HANDBOOK OF CONTRACEPTION AND SEXUAL HEALTH

Offering a comprehensive guide to contraception and sexual health, the new edition of this practical handbook has been fully updated with the latest clinical guidance, research and methods, including new technologies.

Giving clear and detailed information about all contraceptive methods, including how to use them, contra-indications, interactions and common patient anxieties, this guide takes an integrated approach to sexual health. It includes updated chapters on the consultation, person-centred care, anatomy and physiology and sexually transmitted infections. The new edition has been updated and reformatted to increase accessibility.

With plenty of self-assessment exercises, questions and answers and case scenarios, the *Handbook of Contraception and Sexual Health* is an essential read for all nurses, midwives and allied health professionals working in community health and primary care settings.

Suzanne Everett was a senior nurse practitioner in sexual health and worked in sexual health and HIV clinics in London, including the Margaret Pyke Centre, the Camberwell Sexual Health Clinic, the Marlborough Clinic and the Ian Charleson Day Centre until 2023. She was an Associate Professor in sexual health at Middlesex University. She has a PhD that focuses on student nurses' experiences of sexuality in clinical placements. Suzanne is an independent prescriber and worked previously as a practice nurse and nurse specialist in contraceptive and sexual health services, beginning in 1991.

HANDBOOK OF CONTRACEPTION AND SEXUAL HEALTH

FIFTH EDITION

SUZANNE EVERETT

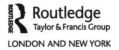

Routledge
Taylor & Francis Group

LONDON AND NEW YORK

Designed cover image: Suzanne Everett

Fifth edition published 2025
by Routledge
4 Park Square, Milton Park, Abingdon, Oxon, OX14 4RN

and by Routledge
605 Third Avenue, New York, NY 10158

*Routledge is an imprint of the Taylor & Francis Group, an informa
business*

First edition published by Baillière Tindall 1998
Fourth edition published by Routledge 2021

British Library Cataloguing-in-Publication Data
A catalogue record for this book is available from the British Library

ISBN: 978-1-032-77705-4 (hbk)
ISBN: 978-1-032-77704-7 (pbk)
ISBN: 978-1-003-48442-4 (ebk)

DOI: 10.4324/9781003484424

Typeset in Sabon
by SPi Technologies India Pvt Ltd (Straive)

Jon and Isobel Everett

CONTENTS

FIGURES

TABLES

ACKNOWLEDGEMENTS

Sexual health is a complex area to work in; we deal with personal issues which often involve abuse and assault. The support from healthcare professionals who work in this area has always been huge, and I would like to thank colleagues who I have worked with at the Ian Charleson Day Centre at Royal Free Hospital and colleagues I have worked with in the past at Marlborough Clinic, Margaret Pyke Centre and Camberwell Sexual Health department.

Huge thanks go to Katie Kinnersley, Jennie Bradford, David Ring, for their continued support and help. Finally, behind every book, I have had huge support from Jon and Isobel.

INTRODUCTION

This book aims to offer a comprehensive introduction to the role of the nurse working in contraception. It addresses some of the problems encountered during consultations and offers the opportunity to test and evaluate your knowledge through self-assessment questions. The answers to these questions are discussed at the end of each chapter.

Sexual health incorporates reproductive sexual health and sexual health. Sexual health as a profession is constantly changing as new methods of contraception become available and as new research is published. All health professionals are accountable for their own actions, and, as management procedures may vary from hospital trusts and GP practices, it is important that you regularly update and understand policies within your workplace, which may be different from this book. It is vital for professionals to keep their knowledge updated. There are several ways to ensure that this happens:

- By becoming an associate member of the College of Sexual and Reproductive Healthcare (Formerly known as the Faculty of Sexual and Reproductive Healthcare) who provides clinical guidance on practice within sexual health, journals and conferences
- By undertaking psychosexual seminar work which involves reflecting on the nurse–client relationship. By looking at the feelings evoked in the nurse–client relationship in this way, problems encountered are seen from a new perspective, helping the nurse's approach to them in the future
- By keeping a reflective diary (Benner, 1994) insight can be gained which may be unavailable if an area is new to a nurse, which can improve future clinical practice

DOI: 10.4324/9781003484424-1

THE CONSULTATION

During a consultation you are in a unique position to give men and women the opportunity to talk about intimate areas of their sexual life and anxieties they may have. However, this will happen only when a client feels they are free to discuss any anxiety or problem. Sometimes clients will give you clues of a problem as they have their hand on the handle of the door and are about to leave the room. Sometimes we miss these clues because we are in a rush or fail to recognise the significance of the clue and only realise its meaning on reflection. In some situations, we may neglect a statement because we have become caught up in our own agenda. Clients may tell you information about themselves which may be upsetting and shocking to you; if your body language, tone of voice or expression shows this, then they will feel that they are unable to disclose any further information for fear of being reproached and judged. It is important never to assume that all clients are heterosexual: reproductive sexual health is not just about preventing pregnancy but also about disease prevention, health promotion and education.

During a consultation, ensure that you are free of interruptions and that total privacy is maintained. Give clients the opportunity to ask questions. Try and ask open-ended questions, for example, "Do you ever have pain or any difficulties during sexual intercourse?" rather than a closed question, such as "You don't have any pain during intercourse?", which only offers the client the opportunity to say "no." Open-ended questions give clients room to bring up problems associated with the area of questioning. Open-ended questions allow clients to express problems which may in fact be commonplace; sometimes clients can feel that they are the only one having difficulties with, for example, a method of contraception, and knowing that they are not alone can be reassuring.

When undertaking any procedure involving a client, it is important to obtain their consent. For a client to give informed consent, you should explain carefully why this procedure is necessary and what it involves. When performing intimate examinations such as vaginal or testicular examinations, you should maintain the client's privacy, allowing them to feel safe without fear of being interrupted by your colleagues or viewed from windows by strangers. Discuss with your client whether they would like a chaperone for any intimate examination.

If you give clients freedom to talk in a non-judgemental environment, then even if they choose not to disclose a problem at an initial consultation, they may return in the future knowing they can feel safe to talk freely.

It is always a good idea to speak to your clients on their own; this ensures that you are gaining their consent and that they are not being coerced into a decision. With young people, this has always been incorporated into the consultation that

DOI: 10.4324/9781003484424-2

at some point, their consultation is on a one-to-one basis. This is to ensure that they are not being groomed or pressurised into sexual intercourse and that you are giving the best possible care with all the information available. Increasingly, all consultations are on a one-to-one basis, and this should be promoted, as clients do not always divulge full information about their sexual histories in front of sexual partners or relatives. By seeing men and women individually, we ensure that a full history is obtained and can address issues of sexual abuse and domestic violence. Relatives who interpret for clients may not fully understand the relevance of questions asked and may not translate all questions and answers completely; as a result, we may not be able to ensure full consent has been obtained from our clients. Following the introduction of the Mental Capacity Act in 2007, it became vital that full consent is gained; to ensure that this happens, qualified interpreters and signers should be used if needed to attain that the client understands and has the mental capacity to consent.

CASE STUDY 1.1

A 34-year-old woman attended with her husband for contraception; the husband walks into the consultation room, and you ask him to wait outside. He appears cross and says his wife wants him in the room; you explain that it is your department's policy* to see clients individually, and he relents and leaves the room. When the woman and you are alone, she says that she did not want him in the room, as he does not want her to use contraception and wants her to get pregnant, which she does not want to do at the moment. You discuss whether she is being emotionally or physically abused, and this does not appear to be the case; you offer help if this changes. You are then able to discuss why she is unable to express herself fully with him and offer contraception.

*(Not all sexual health departments have this policy, so it is important to ascertain what is the practice in your area; if there is not one, you may wish to discuss how you all ensure a complete history has been taken.)

ASSESSMENT

At initial consultations with clients, a full medical history should be taken and updated at regular intervals, which must be dated and documented in the notes for future reference. A complete history includes the general health of the client in the past and present, their gynaecological and sexual health, contraceptive history and the health of their immediate family. Clients can feel threatened by personal questions, especially if they are asked immediately on arrival; try and establish a rapport by finding out the reason for their attendance. Often, by finding out why a client is attending, other questions that you need to know will be answered as a by-product. However, you will need to ask questions which should be open-ended, such as "Do you ever have any pre-menstrual symptoms?", or "Do you ever have migraines?" If a client does have a problem, then you will need to find out more details: for example, if a client has migraines, ask her to describe them and the frequency. You will still need to ask specific questions to eliminate contra-indications to different methods of contraception, such as "When you have a migraine, do you ever see flashing lights or have loss of vision?" Taking a detailed history can take time but can help nurture a good relationship between you and your clients. It can also create the opportunity for them to discuss issues for which insufficient time was given previously.

During the consultation, you should address allergies and medications. Clients often do not consider some over the counter, online and herbal remedies as medications. So, it is important that you really find out what people may be taking, as this may affect the efficacy of the hormonal contraception that is prescribed; an example of this is St John's Wort. Increasingly, men and women are obtaining drugs through the internet, so this is another area you should consider with the people you see.

SEXUAL HISTORY TAKING

Increasingly, contraceptive and genitourinary medicine services are combining or offering similar care to streamline services to clients within sexual health services. With the incidence of sexually transmitted infections rising, it is important to discuss sexually transmitted infections with men and women. Many clients believe that they will know if they become infected, and do not realise that they may be asymptomatic. We should always try to encourage women and their partners to go for screening once they commence a new sexual relationship, and also when they have had unprotected sexual intercourse. As health professionals, we need to be accessible to clients and help empower them with knowledge of sexual health and contraception.

THE CLIENT

Clients who attend for advice on contraception can vary not only in the cultural and religious beliefs they hold but can also have very different attitudes and values about relationships and sexuality. The decisions and problems a client will encounter will depend on where they are in their life: for example, an unplanned pregnancy may be a disaster to a client aged either 15 or 50 for very different reasons, and the decision they make about the pregnancy will be from different perspectives.

Clients who are under 16 years of age may have taken some time to gain enough courage to attend a sexual health clinic and, as a result, may feel embarrassed and awkward. Often, younger clients may attend with a friend, and there may be anxiety over confidentiality, especially if the client is under the age of 16 (see "Confidentiality and Ethics," page 6). They may have already commenced sexual intercourse and require emergency contraception or already be pregnant. Research (Smith, 1993) has shown that the teenage pregnancy rate is higher in deprived areas, but the abortion rate is higher in affluent areas. The abortion rate may be higher in affluent areas for a number of reasons, such as social and parental pressure or that girls from these areas may know how to access abortion services and have the support of their parents. They may have career plans and see a future ahead (Simms, 1993), whilst teenagers living in deprived areas may decide to continue with a pregnancy because of lack of access to abortion services. They may not have career plans and see a pregnancy as their future.

Older men and women are often viewed by society as asexual, and their sexual activity is met with disdain. They may not have discussed intimate areas of their sexual life with anyone and may find the situation embarrassing. Society tends to portray clients over the age of 65 as disinterested in sexual intercourse; however, research shows this is far from the truth. Hinchliff et al.'s (2018) research shows that sexual health is important to older men and women psychologically, socially and physically. Nevertheless, with increasing age, clients may need to adapt their sexual relationship depending on their health and may wish to discuss this. Often, the impact of chronic diseases and medications on sexuality is not fully discussed with clients and their partners. It may take clients some time before they are able to pluck up the courage to discuss these implications or are given the opportunity by professionals to discuss them.

THE NURSE–CLIENT RELATIONSHIP

During a consultation, a relationship develops between the nurse and the client in which feelings and emotions may be expressed. Many clients who consult have no problems and attend for contraceptive advice and supplies; however, other clients may have anxieties and problems that take a great deal of courage to discuss. It is during consultations where there are problems that the recognition of feelings evident within the consultation can help illuminate these problems. This can be sufficient to relieve an anxiety or may bring a hidden problem out into the open where it can be looked at more closely.

Recognising the type of emotion expressed in a consultation can be difficult, and sometimes you may only be able to recognise upon reflection once a client has left. Reflection and psychosexual seminar training can help improve and increase your skills in this area. There are several reasons why we may fail to recognise feelings or acknowledge a problem. Sometimes we lack the confidence to discuss intimate areas with clients and need a great deal of courage to pursue an issue, but this does become easier with practice. On other occasions, our minds may be fixed on our own agenda, which will stop us from listening to the client. For example, there may be a very busy clinic, and you may feel pressurised to "hurry things along," or something the client says may trigger a memory or anxiety in your own personal life. You may have a strong desire "to make things better for the client." However, listening and being there for them is actually what they want, and learning to do this can be difficult initially. There may be occasions when you feel you are not establishing a relationship with the client and are unsure why this is so.

There are several ways to improve your skills in your relationship with your client:

■ Practice listening and recalling conversations. Careful listening can help us pick up clues about how the client feels. Listening will also give you information about the client, which you will need to refer back to, as clients will notice very quickly if you are not listening to what they are talking about.
■ Learn to observe the body language of your clients. You can practice this by watching people around you.
■ What is the client not saying, what are the feelings you are picking up through his/her body language, tone of voice, and facial expression?

- By undertaking Balint seminar training. This is where a group of nurses meet for a set period of time with a seminar leader to discuss the nurse's work. As a group they listen and focus on the feelings invoked by the work; this helps the nurse to look at their work from a new perspective.
- Lastly, a personal reflective diary of your work can help improve your skills.

CONFIDENTIALITY AND ETHICS

All clients have the right to expect that information about themselves or others which is divulged during a consultation will remain confidential. Confidentiality should be respected and only broken in exceptional situations such as if the health, welfare or safety of someone other than the client is at serious risk. If possible, clients should be sensitively encouraged to discuss exceptional areas with people involved themselves. Doctors/nurses who breach confidentiality must be able to show good reason for making this decision (NMC, 2015, updated 2018), which would be an ethical decision. Ethics are the moral code by which a nurse's behaviour is governed within their work with clients and their families and the colleagues they work with.

Clients under the age of 16 are often concerned that any disclosures about their sexual life will be divulged to their parents. This can prevent clients from seeking help with contraception, resulting in unprotected sexual intercourse. Following the Gillick case, the House of Lords (BMA et al., 1993) established that people under the age of 16 are able to give consent to medical treatment regardless of age if they are able to understand what is proposed and the implications and consequences of the treatment. When clients under the age of 16 consult, doctors or nurses should consider the following issues known as the Fraser guidelines:

- The client understands the treatment, its implications and the risks and benefits of it.
- Healthcare professionals should encourage young clients to discuss their consultation with their parents, and their reasons for not wanting to do this. However, confidentiality will still be respected.
- Professionals should consider whether clients are likely to have sexual intercourse without contraception. They should also consider whether the mental and physical health of the client would suffer if the client was not to receive contraception. Lastly, it is important that the client's best interests are taken into account, which may mean giving contraception and advice without parental consent.

GROOMING

"Grooming" is a term used to reflect the befriending of a young or vulnerable person with the purpose of abusing them. This friendship may start online or in person. Groomers who target children through mobile phones and social media now face two years in prison (Gov.UK, 2017). The new "tackling child exploitation support programme" aims to address gang culture, drug dealing, online grooming, sexual exploitation, trafficking and modern slavery and how best to identify and support (GOV.UK, 2019).

Young and vulnerable people who are being groomed often do not realise this is happening to them. During a consultation, you should try to gain a rapport and find out about the person. How did they meet the person they are having sex with? Do they give them expensive gifts? Do they make them do anything they feel uncomfortable with? How old is the person? If they are older by more than five years, then they are in a position of power.

Sometimes you may feel unsure about whether this is a safeguarding issue or not; then, it is always a good idea to talk to adult or child safeguarding teams and your safeguarding lead, and they will be able to advise you. Document all of the information you have collected and any concerns you may have.

It is useful to think about confidentiality as clients (especially young clients) will often be concerned about this area, and you will need to be able to respond to this anxiety sensitively.

Management

Once you have discussed with your client why they have come to see you and have completed a full medical history you will need to address the client's needs. To do this you will need to address their contraceptive and sexual needs using relevant clinical guidance. If a woman cannot have a method of contraception because she has a medical contraindication, you should explain why, so that she understands and is aware of why you cannot give a method of contraception.

If you are not an independent prescriber, you will be working to patient group directives. Whether you are an independent prescriber or work to patient group directives, it is important to understand certain aspects of pharmacology – namely, pharmacokinetics and pharmacodynamics. Pharmacokinetics describes what the body does to the drug, and this includes absorption, distribution, metabolism and elimination of the drug. Pharmacodynamics is about what drugs do to the body; this includes the mechanism of action of the drug and the side effects they can cause. Throughout the hormonal contraceptive chapters, these areas will be addressed. During your assessment of your client, you will be looking for drug interactions, and these can be checked with the British National Formulary and the Faculty of Sexual and Reproductive Healthcare (see other resources at the end of this chapter). One of the most important documents in sexual health is the United Kingdom Medical Eligibility Criteria (UKMEC; FSRH, 2019), which you will need to use in order to prescribe contraception safely. In sexual health, off-label prescribing is quite common and often falls outside patient group directives, but prescribers need to be aware of the guidance surrounding this. You will also hear of quick starting and bridging; terms used when managing women's contraception in complex situations. These terms will be covered in more detail in this chapter.

UNITED KINGDOM MEDICAL ELIGIBILITY CRITERIA (FSRH, 2019)

The United Kingdom Medical Eligibility Criteria (UKMEC) which are based on the World Health guidance for contraception are guidelines are developed and published by the Faculty of Sexual and Reproductive Healthcare. The UKMEC gives clear guidance on whether you can give a method of contraception to someone with a medical condition. It is classified into (Table 1.1):

Table 1.1 United Kingdom Medical Eligibility Criteria (UKMEC; FSRH, 2019)

UKMEC	Guidance
1	A condition where there is no restriction for the use of the contraceptive method.
2	A condition where the advantages of using the method generally outweigh the theoretical or proven risks.
3	A condition where the theoretical or proven risks generally outweigh the advantages of using the method. The provision of a method requires expert clinical judgement and/or referral to a specialist contraceptive provider since use of the method is not usually recommended unless other more appropriate methods are not available or not acceptable.
4	A condition which represents an unacceptable risk if the contraceptive method is used.

Throughout this book, the UKMEC criteria will be referred to highlight conditions where certain methods of contraception are not suitable to be used. The full UKMEC guidelines are available from the Faculty of Sexual and Reproductive Healthcare.

ACTIVITY

Using the UKMEC full guidelines, answer the following questions. You can access the UKMEC guidelines at the Faculty of Sexual and Reproductive Sexual Health website (FSRH) at https://www.fsrh.org/Public/Standards-and-Guidance/uk-medical-eligibility-criteria-for-contraceptive-use-ukmec.aspx.

1. What does the UKMEC say about mild liver cirrhosis and severe cirrhosis and the combined pill? What are the UKMEC categories and the notes about this?
2. What does the UKMEC say about mild liver cirrhosis and severe cirrhosis and the progestogen methods? What are the UKMEC categories?

OFF-LABEL PRESCRIBING

This is where a licenced medication is licenced but used outside its licence. There are many instances where this practice may be advised, one of which is quick starting contraception. There are many more examples where this happens, and prescribers need to be aware of these. Prescribers should be able to justify their practice, and this practice should be supported by published evidence for this indication, and you should be aware that liability sits with the prescriber, the supplier and the dispenser.

QUICK STARTING

This is a practice where clients commence a method of contraception immediately rather than wait to commence with their next period. Quick starting can offer women contraceptive cover faster with no strong adverse effects. Women should always be offered the choice of commencement; if they wish to commence immediately, then pregnancy should be excluded. If pregnancy cannot be excluded, then you should assess the client for emergency contraception and discuss with the client what they would do if they became pregnant. Quick starting can be commenced immediately after levonorgestrel emergency contraception (LNG-EC) onto progestogen pills, combined pills or the progestogen implant is endorsed by the Faculty of Sexual and Reproductive Healthcare if a woman wishes to start immediately and is at continued risk of pregnancy. If a client has ulipristal acetate emergency contraception (UPA-EC), then they should wait five days before commencing hormonal contraception and use barrier contraception in the interim. IUDs, IUS, Co-cyprindiol are not recommended for quick starting (FSRH, 2017b, 2023c). Clients should be advised how long they will need to use alternative contraception when quick starting and the need to perform a pregnancy test in three to four weeks' time to exclude pregnancy.

BRIDGING

If a woman cannot start her chosen method immediately, then she can use a bridging method like the combined methods or progestogen pill until pregnancy has been excluded. A pregnancy test should be performed in three to four weeks' time, and if negative, the chosen method commenced.

USEFUL RESOURCES

Sources of useful information on bridging and quick starting are the Faculty of Sexual and Reproductive Healthcare (www.fsrh.org.uk) and the British Association of Sexual Health and HIV (www.bashh.org.uk), which give guidance on sexually transmitted infections.

If you have a patient who is pregnant or concerned about the effects of medications on pregnancy, the UK Teratology Information Service (www.uktis.org.uk) is a helpful resource.

Information on the safety of medications and drugs can be found from Toxbase, which is the national poisons information service https://wwwtoxbase.org.

2 THE PERSON

Men and women who attend for sexual health services can come with a variety of worries and concerns. The previous chapter discussed consultation; this chapter discusses certain issues that users or patients may attend with. This is not an exclusive list of issues sexual health encompasses such a large area and is complex, so there will always be new issues that arise. At the heart of what we do is the person we see, and it is important to treat everyone as an individual and listen to their anxieties.

YOUNG PEOPLE

The conception rate for women aged under 18 years in England and Wales has more than halved since 2011, when it was 30.9 conceptions per 1,000 women; in 2021, it was 13.2 per 1,000 in women under 18 years (Gov.UK, 2023). This reduction cannot be attributed to one factor, but improved contraceptive use and wider range of choices must have contributed. Young people who become pregnant under the age of 18 are more likely to have poor school attendance and academic progress, and are looked after or leaving care, and are more likely to have experienced a pregnancy previously (NICE, 2019). All methods of contraception should be discussed with all patients, the Faculty of Sexual and Reproductive Healthcare (FSRH) argues that age alone should not limit contraceptive choices (FSRH, 2019a). There has been concern about commencing the injectable Depo-Provera under the age of 18; however, the FSRH, Department of Health, and Medicines and Healthcare Products Regulatory Agency agree that Depo-Provera may be considered in young people under the age of 18 after other methods of contraception have been considered (FSRH, 2019a). This is the result over concerns about bone mass density possibly being reduced in under-18s who have not attained peak bone mass (FSRH, 2019a).

It is important to address safer sex, screening for sexually transmitted infections (STIs) and how to raise these issues with partners with young people. Young people may have a lot of information about STIs or not, so you will need to assess each person individually.

Young people under the age of 16 will need to be assessed against the Fraser guidelines and grooming; this is to ensure that they are not being abused or coerced and are able to consent to treatment (see Chapter 1).

DOI: 10.4324/9781003484424-3

CASE SCENARIO

Mia is 14 years old and attends clinic with her friend Layla, she wants to be seen and is quite nervous and embarrassed. Mia and Layla want to be seen together. You ask Mia to come into your room and explain you will get her friend shortly. Once Mia is sitting down in the consultation room, you explain that you need to ask lots of personal questions about sex. Mia looks embarrassed and says she did not realise this. You go on to explain that whilst it is great to have Layla there in the waiting room, Mia may not want her to know everything about her personal life. Whilst Layla and Mia are friends now, they may not always be, so maybe it is best that she is seen alone. Mia agrees and you see her on her own. As Mia is on her own, you explain about Fraser guidelines. Seeing Mia on her own means that you will get a true picture of what is worrying her, and she will be less likely to modify her story in the presence of her friend.

PORNOGRAPHY

Increasingly young people and men and women are coming into contact with pornography. The children's commissioner and the National Society for the Prevention of Cruelty to Children commissioned research with Middlesex University, which shows young people viewing online pornography both purposefully and inadvertently (Martellozzo et al., 2017). This research reveals the negative effects of porn and how shock and confusion can dissipate with users becoming desensitised to the content (Martellozzo et al., 2017). The author has experienced student nurses on wards encountering male patients accessing pornography on the wards on their phones. Staff have lacked experience on how to address the situation. This highlights the need to discuss pornography with patients and to train staff in how to discuss and address this area.

LEARNING DISABILITIES

Men and women who have learning disabilities are vulnerable to being groomed; are more likely to live in poverty, have poor health, and suffer from loneliness; and are likely to be the victims of discrimination and bullying. Patients with learning disabilities may find it harder to access healthcare and, when they access it, find it difficult to communicate and understand issues related to health. This may mean that they are more at risk of STIs and pregnancy. They are more likely to be isolated and discriminated against and may have poor housing and be unemployed. People with learning disabilities are vulnerable to the crime called "cuckooing," which is where a drug dealer grooms a vulnerable person and then takes over their home and uses it to produce drugs. Healthcare professionals need to gain the trust of learning disability patients so that a relationship can be established; this involves adult safeguarding teams to support communication across healthcare teams.

National Health Services (NHS) England advocates that the following key points are addressed when assessing people with learning disabilities.

- Awareness by healthcare professionals of misattributing symptoms to a person's learning disability leading to mismanagement (i.e., diagnostic overshadowing).
- Use of healthcare passports, if the person has one, to aid communication.
- Assess each person individually.
- Listen to parents and carers.
- Make reasonable adjustments.
- Communicate with the person.
- Understand that responses to pain and discomfort may be different.
- Awareness of the Mental Capacity Act.
- Utilise the support of the learning disability team.
- Further training or eLearning on the Oliver McGowan Mandatory Training on Learning Disability and Autism.
- Awareness of mental well-being and the increased incidence of mental health problems and how you can support the person to reduce these.

(NHS England, 2023)

DOMESTIC ABUSE

Domestic violence is any "incident or a pattern of incidents of controlling, coercive, threatening behaviour, violence or abuse between those aged 16 or over who are, or have been, intimate partners or family members regardless of gender or sexuality" (RCN, 2020a).

Domestic violence can be physical, emotional, psychological, financial, sexual and coercive. Domestic violence is not gender specific. It can happen over a long period of time or be a one-off episode. Like female genital mutilation (FGM) it is important to ask all patients if they have experienced domestic violence; this gives everyone the opportunity to voice concerns. Nowadays, asking about domestic violence is usually on a list of compulsory questions we ask in sexual health. Patients have often said that they were victims of domestic violence in the past, but no one asked them at the time, and if asked, this may have encouraged them to voice concerns. So, it is important that we do not neglect this area.

Domestic abuse can take many forms, and these may include the following:

- Physical abuse
- Psychological or emotional abuse, including gaslighting
- Sexual abuse
- Financial abuse
- Coercive and controlling behaviour
- Online abuse
- Harassment or stalking
- "Honour"-based abuse
- Forced marriage
- FGM

(RCN, 2023)

CASE SCENARIO

J is an 18-year-old man who attends with dysuria; during the consultation, he reveals to Kate, the nurse, that he is sleeping on his friend's sofa. Kate asks why he is doing this, and he reveals that his father used to beat him up, and the police intervened and advised him to leave home. He does not have any money and is finishing his "A" levels. Kate contacts adult safeguarding teams in ManKind, a charity for men who are victims of domestic violence, at https://mankind. org.uk/.

Domestic abuse highlights the importance of seeing patients on their own. If you see a client with a member of their family, it is possible that they are the perpetrator of the abuse, and your client will not be able to talk to you about it. Victims of abuse may have intrusive people trying to attend consultations as well, who may be aggressive or dominant or over-attentive. The victim may appear submissive and afraid to speak up with their abuser present.

Signs of domestic abuse (RCN, 2020a)

- Depression
- Anxiety
- Alcohol or substance misuse
- Self-harming or suicidal tendencies
- Missed appointments, attending with vague symptoms at appointments or repeated appointments
- Non-compliance with medical treatment
- Injuries inconsistent with history, multiple injuries
- Unexplained gastrointestinal symptoms or genitourinary symptoms
- Long-term pain, long-term pelvic pain or dyspareunia
- Unintended pregnancy
- Delayed antenatal care, history of premature labour or stillbirths
- Vaginal bleeding or recurring STIs or urinary tract infections (UTIs)
- Neglect
- Headaches, cognitive problems, hearing loss
- Victims of the abuse may blend into the background and appear normal, not wanting to draw attention to their situation

Clients may or may not have the above signs of domestic abuse. Taking time to listen to the person and what is going on in their lives will help create a rapport. If they are not ready at their first visit to divulge the abuse, they may come back and tell you; creating trust will encourage this. If a patient is a victim of domestic abuse, you should contact child or adult safeguarding (depending on their age) and your safeguarding lead.

Resources

- The government website contains useful resources on domestic violence https://www.gov.uk/government/publications/domestic-abuse-act-2021/ domestic-abuse-statutory-guidance-accessible-version
- National Domestic Abuse helpline run by Refuge – Freephone 24 hour: 0808 2000 247. British Sign Language access from 10 am to 6 pm on weekdays. The website offers a live chat service between 3pm and 10pm on weekdays

FEMALE GENITAL MUTILATION

Women who have had FGM may describe themselves as victims or survivors of this practice. They may refer to FGM, or *Sunna* or cutting (RCN, 2016, updated 2023). Some women may not even know whether they have experienced FGM because they were very young or have locked this memory away. But the long-term consequences of this practice are huge and can be devastating.

As part of mandatory reporting, we need to ask all women about whether they know about FGM and have experienced it (Home Office, 2020). You might want to ask, "Do you know what FGM is?" and then follow this with, "Have you ever been cut?" It is important to ask all women because this will raise awareness but also there is an assumption that FGM is only performed in certain countries, and if we only ask women of a certain country, we will miss women from other countries who have experienced it. It is important to not make assumptions and ask all women. Whilst FGM is found in 27 African countries, it is also found in Asia and the Middle East (e.g. Yemen, Iraq), and amongst diaspora communities worldwide (Home Office, 2020).

MANDATORY REPORTING

Mandatory reporting was introduced in 2015 with the Serious Crime Act (RCN, 2016, updated 2023). This means that all regulated health, social care and teaching professionals must report cases of FGM in girls under the age of 18 years to the police. This professional duty cannot be transferred to anyone else (RCN, 2016, updated 2023). If a girl under 18 years old is at immediate risk of FGM, then the police should be rung on 999, and as this is only one part of safeguarding, the safeguarding lead will need to be involved. If you observe or a girl under 18 years tells you that she has had FGM and is not in immediate danger, then you will need to report it to the police on telephone 101, and child safeguarding procedures will need to be followed. A map of FGM reporting procedures is available at the Department of Health (Home Office, 2020).

If a woman has had FGM and is over the age of 18, the police do not need to be informed. However, if she has children under the age of 18 years old, then safeguarding procedures will need to be followed, as they may be at risk of FGM from family or relatives.

> Under the Serious Crime Act in 2015 and the Female Genital Mutilation Act 2003 not only is FGM illegal in England and Wales. It is an offence to fail to protect a girl from the risk of FGM (HM Government. 2016). There is extra-territorial jurisdiction over offences of FGM committed abroad by UK

nationals and permanent residents, and FGM protection orders can be used
to protect girls at risk.

15

The person

(HM Government, 2016)

WHY DOES FGM HAPPEN?

There are many reasons why FGM occurs, and whilst it is illegal in the UK, parents may come under pressure from family and members of their community either in the UK or abroad to have FGM performed on their daughters. Some of the reasons why FGM is performed are to curb sexuality and increase marriageability, to preserve a girl's cultural identity. FGM may be upheld as a religious obligation by some Muslim populations, even though the practice predates Islam, and it is practised by Muslims, Christians and followers of traditional African religions alike (RCN, 2016, updated 2023).

TYPES OF FGM

The subdivisions of types I to III are to help when documenting types of FGM. However, it is difficult sometimes to classify the type of FGM, as this may have been done a long time ago and pubic hair growth can make identification harder. The World Health Organization classification of the types of FGM is used for identification (WHO, 2024; Table 2.1).

Table 2.1 Classification of FGM (WHO, 2024)

Classification	Description
Type 1	This is the partial or total removal of the clitoral glans (the external and visible part of the clitoris, which is a sensitive part of the female genitals), and/or the prepuce/clitoral hood (the fold of skin surrounding the clitoral glans).
Type 2	This is the partial or total removal of the clitoral glans and the labia minora (the inner folds of the vulva), with or without removal of the labia majora (the outer folds of skin of the vulva).
Type 3	Also known as infibulation, this is the narrowing of the vaginal opening through the creation of a covering seal. The seal is formed by cutting and repositioning the labia minora, or labia majora, sometimes through stitching, with or without removal of the clitoral prepuce/clitoral hood and glans.
Type 4	This includes all other harmful procedures to the female genitalia for non-medical purposes, e.g. pricking, piercing, incising, scraping and cauterising the genital area.

RISKS OF FGM

The short-term and long-term implications of FGM are severe. This is a practice which is not discussed amongst women who have had FGM, and so they are often unaware of its long-term consequences.

- Haemorrhage, pain shock, wound infection, septicaemia, tetanus
- Urine retention, pelvic infection
- Injury to other tissues, e.g. vaginal fistulae
- Ulceration of genital region
- Risk of bacterial, hepatitis B or HIV infection due to instruments being re-used without sterilisation
- Post-traumatic stress disorder
- Infertility from pelvic infection and obstructed genital tract
- Traumatic intercourse, obstructed labour
- Recurrent UTIs can lead to kidney failure
- Death

SUPPORTING WOMEN WITH FGM

Women who have experienced FGM may find it difficult to have penetrative sexual intercourse and as a result may find it difficult to get pregnant. Women who have had FGM and are pregnant need to be assessed. Depending on the type of FGM, deinfibulation may need to be performed as the vaginal orifice may be too small to allow progression of the foetus during labour. This is not a reversal of FGM procedures as it is not possible to reverse the damage of FGM. Deinfibulation is best performed before 20 weeks of gestation; this reduces the risk of cutting stretched scar tissue in labour and further damage (RCN, 2016, updated 2023). Deinfibulation will also ensure that the woman will be able to empty her bladder; this is important in normal delivery and caesarean sections. Deinfibulation should be carried out by an experienced and trained healthcare professional.

Women who are experiencing problems following FGM and not pregnant should be referred to gynaecology related to infertility, menorrhagia or difficulties having penetrative sexual intercourse. Counselling may be needed for the woman and her partner. Men can be traumatised by the effects of FGM and can be horrified by the damage done to their partners.

Gender

There are lots of different terms now, and these can be confusing. If a patient you are seeing uses terms you are unsure about, be honest and ask them to explain.

Gender terms definitions:

- Gender binary = identified as male or female
- Binary = identify by the sex/gender from birth
- Non-binary = is where people do identify as male or female
- Cisgender = this is where an individual's gender matched their assignment at birth
- Affirmed gender = a person's gender achieved after transition
- Assignment at birth = someone's sex identified and registered at birth

TRANSSEXUAL PERSON

The term "transsexual" refers to a person who does not identify with the sex they were born with. Transsexual people experience a gender identity that is inconsistent with, or not culturally associated with, their assigned sex. They desire to permanently transition to the gender with which they identify, usually seeking medical assistance (including hormone replacement therapy and other sex reassignment therapies).

They have often spent several years trying to gain help, and many have had mental health issues over their journey; they may feel that they would rather die than live in the body that they have been born with. Health professionals can lack training and knowledge in this area and feel unequipped to help trans men and trans women. Trans men and trans women may meet discrimination from health professionals and patients who feel that they should not share the same toilets or wards. It is important that as health professionals we look after all patients equally, and these men and women will need a lot of support and sensitivity (RCN, 2020b).

Trans men and women may attend services with little information, so it is important that we ask all patients about medical history and medications.

TRANSGENDER PERSON

Transgender people have a gender identity or gender expression that differs from their assigned sex. Transgender people are sometimes called transsexual if they desire medical assistance to transition from one sex to another.

GENDER REASSIGNMENT SURGERY

Sex reassignment surgery, or SRS (also known as gender reassignment surgery, gender confirmation surgery, genital reconstruction surgery, gender-affirming surgery or sex realignment surgery), is the surgical procedure (or procedures) by which a transsexual person's physical appearance and function of their existing sexual characteristics are altered to resemble that which is associated with that gender.

TRANSGENDER MEN

A transgender man or trans man will originally be born a woman and will have to live as a man for a year prior to surgery. He will need to take masculinising hormone therapy which can produce side effects such as increased risk of polycythaemia and venous thromboembolism, increased cholesterol and liver function abnormalities (Gupta, 2016; RCN, 2020b). The testosterone administration will stop menstruation rapidly and supress ovarian function. Trans men are recommended to have a hysterectomy to prevent endometrial hyperplasia. If a trans man does not have a hysterectomy, maybe because he wants to have a baby, then he should be advised to have ultrasounds every two years for endometrial hyperplasia screening (RCN, 2020b). Trans men who have retained their uterus and cervix will share the same risk of cervical cancer as women do, and the need to have cervical screening should be discussed. Trans men who have had breast reduction have a lower risk of breast cancer but there may be breast tissue, and breast awareness should be encouraged, and future breast screening should be encouraged.

If a trans man needs to be catheterised, then it will need to be based on their genital presentation; trans men with a phalloplasty can be catheterised the same as other men. A phalloplasty is a construction or reconstruction of a penis using veins and arteries from forearm or thigh to create a graft and shaft of the penis. A metoidioplasty is the creation of a penis and scrotum done by cutting the ligament surrounding the clitoris to create these.

TRANS MEN AND CONTRACEPTION AND SEXUAL HEALTH

Trans men who have received gonadotrophin releasing hormone analogues to supress ovarian function should be warned that they cannot rely on this for contraception. Contraception is advised if a trans man has not had a hysterectomy and is having vaginal sex and does not want to get pregnant (FSRH, 2017). All contraceptive methods are suitable depending on their medical health (FSRH, 2017). Trans men who are taking testosterone should be warned that this is teratogenic if they become pregnant (FSRH, 2017). Trans men should be considered for human papillomavirus (HPV) vaccination to reduce the risk of HPV-associated cancers.

TRANSGENDER WOMAN

A transgender woman or trans woman will originally be born a man and will have to live as a woman for a year prior to surgery. Trans women will be given feminising hormone therapy that can produce side effects that include increased liver function abnormalities, increase in venous thromboembolism and increase in hyperprolactinaemia (RCN, 2020b). Feminising hormone therapy can increase the risk of osteoporosis and breast cancer in some trans women (RCN, 2020b). Trans women should be shown how to be breast aware and advised about the risks of osteoporosis and how to reduce this.

Trans women can have a vaginoplasty, which is the creation of a vagina and vulva; this includes mons pubis, labia, clitoris and urethra. Trans women can be catheterised the same as other women. Trans women who have a vaginoplasty are required to dilate their vaginas regularly. It is suggested that this be three times a day for eight weeks and then twice daily afterwards (RCN, 2020b), eventually reducing to once a week, but this will need to be continued throughout life (RCN, 2020b). Trans women will be taught how to do this. Some trans women will undergo labiaplasty rather than a vaginoplasty which is the creation of a labia, but no vagina will be created. To create breasts, trans women may have breast augmentation surgery.

TRANS WOMEN AND CONTRACEPTION AND SEXUAL HEALTH

Trans women who have not undergone an orchidectomy (removal of the testicles) or vasectomy (male sterilisation) need to be aware that if they have vaginal sex, there is a risk of pregnancy. Oestradiol therapy can result in impaired spermatogenesis, and gonadotrophin releasing hormone analogues, finasteride and cyproterone

Table 2.2 Screening of trans men and trans women (Gov.UK, 2023)

Screening test	Trans women	Trans men
Breast screening	Yes	Yes, if they have breast tissue present
Cervical screening	No	Yes, if they have not had a hysterectomy and have a cervix
Abdominal aortic aneurysm screening	Yes	No
Bowel screening	Yes	Yes
Prostate screening	Yes, if the prostate gland is still present.	No
HPV screening	Yes	Yes

acetate can reduce or block sperm production, but they should not be relied on as contraceptive protection (FSRH, 2017).

If a trans woman experiences vaginal bleeding, it is not normal in trans women, and if it is not related to post-operative recovery, it should be investigated immediately. Not all gender reassignment procedures involve removing the prostate, so these trans women will be at risk of prostate cancer and need to be aware of screening as they get older (Gov.UK, 2023; Table 2.2).

Issues that need to be considered in care of trans men and trans women

- Healthcare needs to be individualised.
- Don't make assumptions about your patients' sexuality and the gender of their partner.
- How much do you need to know? Is your question relevant to your work? Are you being nosey?
- We need to ask about medications with all patients, over the counter, recreational and herbal remedies. All patients can self-medicate with medicines sourced from the internet, and trans men and women are a high risk for this.
- As with all patients, think about their mental health, ask about domestic violence, is there any abuse? Are they being groomed? Are they vulnerable?

ACTIVITY

Do you still have questions that have not been answered? Try looking at the Stonewall website at the Truth about Trans (stonewall.org.uk).

THE OLDER CLIENT

It is often assumed that as men and women get older, they will be disinterested in sexual intercourse, and they will not be having sexual intercourse. This assumption means that older men and women do not get asked about any problems or that health professionals do not address the effects of age and illness on people's abilities to have sexual intercourse. Chapter 3 discusses the changes in anatomy and physiology with age in men and women. Older patients may feel embarrassed accessing sexual health services; they may feel that they should not have made mistakes at their age, e.g. requiring emergency contraception. Hinchliff et al.'s research shows increasing evidence that sexual health is important to older men and women psychologically, socially and physically, and highlights how important it is for health professionals to recognise these needs (Hinchliff et al., 2018).

Illness and sexuality

Acute and long-term medical conditions can affect the ability to have sexual intercourse. Health professionals often do not address this issue; this can be because of time constraints or because the health professional is embarrassed or feels ill-equipped to answer questions this may provoke.

Healthcare is managed in asexual manner with the perception that sexual concerns are unimportant patients are often expected to meet professionals' perspective of the sick role, yet if you are seriously ill, sexual contact may be even more important. The way we as health professionals avoid addressing this area is through lack of education and focusing on the medical condition. It is important that health professionals address the effects of medication and surgical intervention on the ability to have sexual intercourse so that patients are fully informed and able to give consent. We need to be aware of our patients' sexual needs and be able to address these and listen to their anxieties.

ACTIVITY

- Do you know if any of the medications or medical treatments you use affect erectile function?
- Do you know where your patients can get help for erectile dysfunction? Try and find out what local resources are available.

Further reading and resources

- The Beaumont Society – a national self-help body (www.beaumontsociety. org.uk)
- National Domestic Abuse Helpline 0808 2000 247. 24-hour freephone
- DEPEND – advice and support for family members and partners (www. depend.org.uk)
- The Gender Trust – support for those affected by gender identity issues (www. gendertrust.org.uk)
- Mermaids – support for families, children and young people with gender identity issues (www.mermaidsuk.org.uk)
- FGM help – fgmhelp@nspcc.org.uk or telephone: 0800 028 3550
- LGBT health and well-being – www.lgbthealth.org.uk

- GIRES – Gender Information Research and Education Society – aims to improve outcomes for people and also keeps a local and national support directory (www.gires.org.uk)
- ManKind Initiative – www.mankind.org.uk
- TranzWiki – www.TranzWiki.net
- Royal College of Nursing – www.rcn.org.uk/clinical-topics/domestic-violence-and-abuse

3

ANATOMY AND PHYSIOLOGY

INTRODUCTION

The male and female reproductive systems are important for procreation, the creation of offspring. They can be used to allow expression of sexual desires and emotional intimacy; they can adversely be used to exert power and inflict violence. Understanding the anatomy and physiology of these systems and the influence of hormones is vital for professionals working in sexual health areas to be able to differentiate between normal and abnormal. For example, understanding the difference between physiological discharge and pathological discharge is a useful tool to use when educating women on fertility awareness or when discussing vaginal infections such as bacterial vaginosis.

Exercise

You may find it useful to continue your reading after this chapter with Chapter 4, "Fertility Awareness."

MALE REPRODUCTION SYSTEM

The male reproductive system includes the **penis** and two **testes**. The testes are located in the **scrotum**. The scrotum consists of skin and subcutaneous tissue (Figures 3.1–3.3).

A vertical septum of subcutaneous tissue divides it into two parts, each containing one testis. There are approximately 500 seminiferous tubules per testis. The tubules are divided by fibrous septae and surrounded by the **tunica albuginea**. Each tubule is 30–70 cm long. The location of the testes, outside the abdominal cavity, provides a temperature about 3°C below normal body temperature. This lower temperature is necessary for production of viable sperm. Interstitial tissue between the **seminiferous tubules** contains connective tissue, blood vessels, lymphatics and **Leydig cells** which produce **testosterone**. In each testis there are tubules and ducts which form the **epididymis**, which then leads on to become the **vas deferens**, which enlarges to become the **ampulla**. The **seminal vesicle** joins each vas deferens at the lower end of the ampulla; these tubes then become known as the ejaculatory ducts. The ejaculatory ducts then fuse to the urethra in the **prostate gland** to become one duct, the prostatic urethra. The **prostatic urethra** will then carry semen and urine, the **bulbourethral glands** (Cowper's gland) join the **urethra**, which enters the **penis**. The penis comprises three

DOI: 10.4324/9781003484424-4

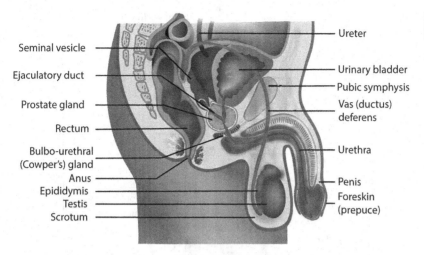

Figure 3.1 Sagittal section of the male reproductive organs.

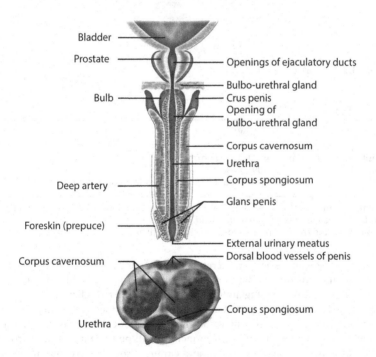

Figure 3.2 Internal male reproductive system.

cylindrical bodies: two dorsal corpora cavernosa and one corpus spongiosum. The urethra ends at the **external urethral meatus**. The head of the penis is usually covered by **prepuce** or **foreskin**, which can be removed in circumcision.

The seminal vesicles, prostate gland and bulbourethral glands are all accessory sex glands which provide sperm with transport medium and nutrients (Table 3.1).

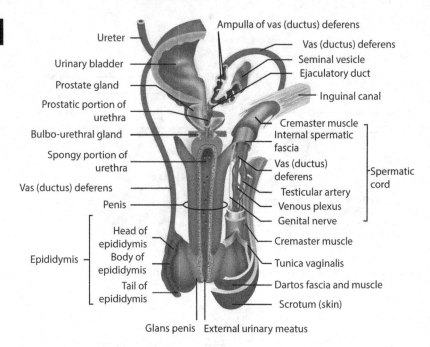

Figure 3.3 Sagittal section of the penis.

Table 3.1 Composition of semen

Volume of ejaculate	2–6 ml*
Density of spermatozoa	60–150 million/ml
Morphology	60%–80% normal shape
Motility	50% should be motile after incubation for one hour at 37°C

Semen, or seminal fluid, consists of spermatozoa and secretions from the bulbourethral glands, seminal vesicles and prostate gland.
* Values outside these normal ranges indicate infertility.

The seminal vesicles – These are secretory glands found in the base of the prostate gland and provide the transport medium for sperm. The fluid is alkaline and contains fructose, prostaglandins, ascorbic acid and globulins.

The prostate gland – This is found in the neck of the bladder in an adult; it is 3 cm in diameter and contains mucosal glands. Prostatic secretions are thin and milky and contain enzymes, which include acid phosphatase, acid hydrolase, protease, fibrinolysin and calcium and citrates. Prostate secretions are important for stimulating sperm motility and for neutralising vaginal acidity.

The bulbourethral glands – These secrete mucus to provide lubrication during ejaculation; they are found between the prostate and the penis.

MALE HORMONES

Three hormones are the principal regulators of the male reproductive system: hypothalamic hormone, anterior pituitary hormones and testicular hormones.

Anterior pituitary hormones control spermatogenesis and androgen production, and these are called the follicle-stimulating hormone or the luteinizing hormone.

Follicle-stimulating hormone (FSH) stimulates spermatogenesis by acting on the seminiferous tubules.

Luteinizing hormone (LH), also known as **interstitial cell-stimulating hormone (ICSH)**, is required for completion of spermatogenesis by stimulating production of androgens in the interstitial cells of the Leydig cells.

Testosterone stimulates the development of male secondary sex characteristics and spermatogenesis. Ninety-five per cent of testosterone is synthesised and stored in the interstitial cells in the testes and 5% is produced in the adrenal glands. Testosterone is synthesised from cholesterol, and the total adult male level is 12–30 nmol 1^{-1}. It is circulated in the plasma targeting reproductive organs and somatic tissues, which produce the male physique, stimulation epiphyseal growth, growth of facial and body hair, libido, lowering of voice, increase in sebum secretion and mild electrolyte retention. Testosterone is metabolised and excreted by the liver.

Inhibin is thought to be produced by the Sertoli cells in response to FSH stimulation and exerts negative feedback on FSH release.

PRODUCTION OF SPERM

Production of sperm, called **spermatogenesis**, happens in the seminiferous tubules in the **testes**. The **seminiferous tubules** are surrounded by a connective tissue which contains **Leydig cells** (interstitial cells), which are responsible for synthesis and production of male hormones. In the seminiferous, there are **germ cells** and **Sertoli cells**. Some of the germ cells mature to become **primary spermatocytes**. The primary spermatocytes undergo meiotic division to become **secondary spermatocytes**. These then undergo further meiotic division to become **spermatids**. **Spermatids** transform into **spermatozoa** with the support from Sertoli cells, which it is attached to; it is thought that Sertoli cells help with nutrition of germ cells. Once the **spermatozoa** have been produced, they are released from **Sertoli cells** into the **lumen** of the **seminiferous tubules**. It takes 70–100 days for production of mature sperm.

Once the **spermatozoa** are fully formed, they are pushed along the **seminiferous tubules** into the head of the **epididymis**. The tail of the epididymis is the main storage area for spermatozoa. A storage area is important, as the process of spermatogenesis is continuous, whilst ejaculations occur at intervals, so the spermatozoa need a storage area until it is needed, which can be up to 42 days. If ejaculation does not occur, the spermatozoa degenerate. Mature spermatozoa move from the epididymis into the **vas deferens** and join the seminal vesicle and the **ejaculatory duct**. The vas deferens is made of connective tissue and three layers of smooth muscle and autonomic nerve supply. This gives the vas deferens the ability to contract quickly during ejaculation. It is this peristaltic wave and spermatozoa's ability to swim that allow sperm to be released through the urethra during ejaculation.

FEMALE REPRODUCTION SYSTEM

There are 400 ova released over a female's reproductive life of 30–40 years. Menarche is the commencement of the menstrual cycle and usually starts around the age of 12–13 but can be between 9 and 17 years. The production of ova occurs in the **ovaries,** of which there are two; they have an irregular outer shape and are 4 cm long, 2 cm wide and 1 cm thick (Figures 3.4 and 3.5).

The outer surface is made of columnar cells called **germinal epithelium.** The next layer is called the **tunica albuginea** made of fibrous connective tissue; this is followed by the cortex, where **female germ cells** are located which become oocytes; finally, the inner layer is called the **vascular medulla.**

Follicles are developing oocyte and follicular tissue. The **primordial follicle** comprises cuboidal cells, which divide to form **granulosa cells.** Outside the follicle, the interstitial cells change and become the **theca folliculi;** the inner layer of this produces **oestrogens.** The follicle increases in size and becomes the **secondary follicle.** The secondary follicle matures, and the **granulosa cells** split to form the **corona radiata** around the oocyte, and the outer layer forms the **membrane granulosa.** This becomes the **Graafian follicle,** which moves the surface of the ovary.

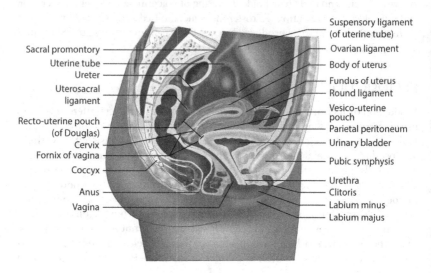

Figure 3.4 Sagittal section of the female reproductive organs.

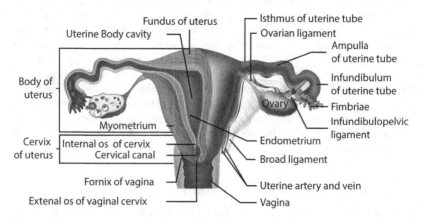

Figure 3.5 Internal female reproductive system.

A mature ovum develops within the follicle, the primordial germ cells differentiate into oogonia, and by 12 weeks of intrauterine life, they have undergone mitotic division to produce primary oocytes.

Ovulation is the release of the ovum from the Graafian follicle; it is thought that the follicular fluid pressure increases, causing the release of the ovum. **Inhibin** has been found in follicular fluid, and it is thought that this may determine how many follicles are released at ovulation and may have links with polycystic ovary disease. Anovulation occurs in 10% of ovarian cycles, but if women have regular menstrual cycles, this indicates ovulation. Some women experience lower abdominal pain on ovulation, which is known as mittelschmerz, and some may experience a small amount of bleeding, which is due to falling hormone levels.

The collapsed follicle becomes the **corpus luteum**, which secretes oestrogen and progesterone for maintaining a pregnancy if this occurs until 12 weeks; after this time, the placenta takes over this role. If there is no pregnancy, the corpus luteum will degenerate after 12–14 days, becoming the **corpus albicans**. If fertilisation occurs, it happens in the ampulla of the **fallopian tube** or **uterine tube**. Only one spermatozoon can enter one ovum. There are two uterine tubes that lie within the folds of the **broad ligament**; each tube is 10–15 cm in length and is divided into four parts.

Interstitial portion joins the wall of the uterus, whilst the **isthmus** is next and slightly wider, followed by the **ampulla**, which is the widest part of the uterine tube and where fertilisation occurs, and finally, the **infundibulum** is trumpet shaped and has fimbria that are attached to the ovary. The uterine tube has three layers, is covered by **peritoneum** and has a thin **muscular layer** followed by a **serous layer** of ciliated columnar epithelium, which wafts the ovum from the infundibulum to the uterus. This serous layer has many folds called plicae and goblet-shaped cells which produce secretions to provide nutrition to the ovum.

The fertilised ovum enters the **uterus** five to six days after ovulation and four days after fertilisation, and it embeds in the endometrium, where it will continue to grow and develop as the foetus. The uterus is pear shaped and consists of two parts: the **corpus**, or **body**, and the **cervix**. The **body** is the upper two thirds and is 5 cm long and is usually anteverted and anteflexed, which means it is tilted forwards. The **fundus** is the uppermost rounded aspect of the uterus and lies above where the uterine tubes are inserted; this area is called the **cornua**. The isthmus is 7 mm and is situated at the junction of the uterus and the cervix. The wall of the uterus is made of three layers: the inner layer is the **endometrium**; the middles muscular layer is called the **myometrium**; the outer cover of the peritoneum is called the **perimetrium**. The uterus has three important functions: firstly, to receive the ovum; secondly, to provide an environment for the growth and development of the foetus; and, finally, to expel the foetus and placenta when the pregnancy is complete.

The **cervix** is at the lowest end of the uterus and is 2.5 cm in length; the lower end projects into the vagina. In the cavity of the cervix, there is an **internal os**, which communicates to the uterus, and the **external os**, which communicates to the vagina.

The **vagina** is a fibromuscular tube which is directed backwards and upwards; it extends from the cervix to the vulva and has the ability to expand to allow a fully grown foetus through. The anterior wall of the vagina is shorter and 7.5 cm in length, whilst the posterior wall is longer and 10 cm in length (Figure 3.6).

The vagina is kept lubricated by secretions from the cervical glands and transudation of serous fluid from blood vessels on the surface. The vaginal fluid has a

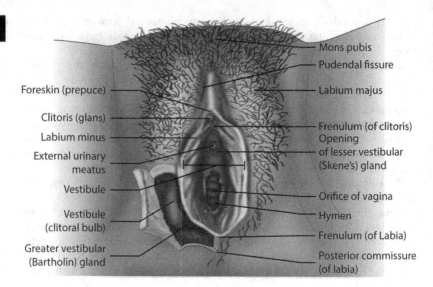

Mons pubis
Pudendal fissure
Foreskin (prepuce)
Labium majus
Clitoris (glans)
Labium minus
Frenulum (of clitoris)
Opening
of lesser vestibular
(Skene's) gland
External urinary
meatus
Vestibule
Orifice of vagina
Vestibule
(clitoral bulb)
Hymen
Frenulum (of Labia)
Greater vestibular
(Bartholin) gland
Posterior commissure
(of labia)

Figure 3.6 External female genitalia.

pH of 4.5 and contains lactic acid, and this is produced by lactobacilli working on the glycogen in the squamous cells of the vaginal lining. This lactic acid helps destroy any bacteria which enter the vagina.

The vagina opens to the vaginal orifice or introitus and the **external genitalia**. The vaginal orifice lies between the labia minora and the urethra, and is partially occluded by the **hymen**. The hymen is a thin membrane; in a virgin, someone who has not had sexual intercourse, it is intact and has a small opening. Following first sexual intercourse, this is ruptured, and after vaginal delivery, it is torn further, leaving a small amount of tissue and is known as carunculae myrtiformes. **Bartholin's glands** lie on either side of the vagina and open into the vaginal canal and their secretions along with **Skene's glands** lubricate the vulva and are increased in response to the erection of the **clitoris**, helping to facilitate vaginal intercourse. Skene's glands are located behind the urethral meatus. The **urethral meatus** is the opening below the clitoris from where the urethral canal begins. The **vestibule** is the area which contains the vagina and urethra and is only seen when the **labia minora** is separated. The clitoris is 2.5 cm long and contains erectile tissue and is found at the junction of the labia minora (Figure 3.7).

It contains two erectile bodies – the **corpora cavernosa** and the **glans clitoris**, which when stimulated become erect and fill with blood just like the penis.

Labia minora are two folds of skin that encircle the clitoris, forming a **hood** or **prepuce**, and then divide to enclose the vestibule and finishes as a thin fold of skin known as the **fourchette**. The **labia majora** are two thick folds of fatty tissue which extend from the **mons veneris** to the perineal body. The inner surface is smooth, and the outer surface is covered by hair. The **mons veneris** is a pad of fat over the pubic bone and is covered by skin and hair.

It is important for a health professionals to know what the normal external genitalia looks like, and that when a woman is examined vaginally this area is observed to ensure that any abnormalities are detected.

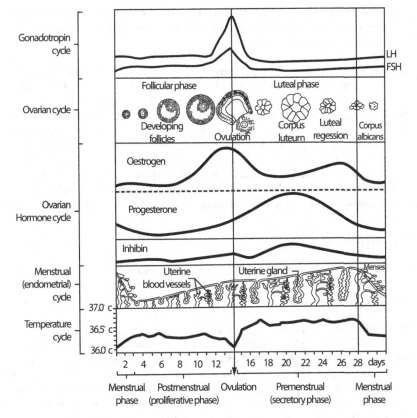

Figure 3.7 Female reproductive cycle.

The menstrual cycle is usually 28 days but can vary between 21 and 35 days. It is divided into the follicular and luteal phases. The follicular phase is when the follicle matures and ruptures, and the luteal phase is the formation of the corpus luteum, its development and degeneration.

FEMALE HORMONES

There are four main hormones which are the principal regulators of the female reproductive system.

- **Follicle-stimulating hormone** (FSH) stimulates follicle development and oestrogen production.
- **Luteinizing hormone** (LH) stimulates the release of the ovum.
- **Oestrogen** prepares the body and uterus for ovulation and pregnancy. It is responsible for the growth of the body, sex organs, secondary sex characteristics, prepares the endometrium for pregnancy, makes cervical mucus thinner and more alkaline.
- **Progesterone** prepares the body for pregnancy by maintaining the endometrium when pregnancy occurs. It stimulates the development of lobules and

alveoli in the mammary glands. Premenstrual water retention is attributed to progesterone, and it causes a slight rise in basal body temperature during the luteal phase following ovulation.

Following menstruation, there are **low levels of oestrogen;** the hypothalamus detects this and **increases GnRH,** which causes **FSH to be increased.** FSH stimulates follicle development, which **increases oestrogen production.** The **higher levels of oestrogen** are detected by the hypothalamus, **which reduces FSH levels.** Oestrogen prepares the uterus and body for ovulation. Because of the **high levels of oestrogen** there is **positive feedback** to the hypothalamus where upon production of **LH, ovulation occurs.** The corpus luteum forms from the collapsed follicle after ovulation and secretes progesterone and oestrogen; these stop gonadotrophins and prepare the body for pregnancy. If the ovum is **not fertilised,** then the corpus luteum degenerates, hormone levels drop and menstruation occurs.

The menstrual cycle

The menstrual cycle describes the changes to the endometrium. The menstrual cycle is usually 28 days in length but can vary between 21 and 35 days. The menstrual cycle is divided into three stages:

The **proliferative phase** lasts 10–11 days and coincides with ovarian follicle growth and secretion of oestrogen. The endometrium gradually builds up.
The **secretory phase** lasts for 14 days and is under the influence of progesterone and oestrogens. The endometrium is now 5 mm in thickness. If after 12–14 days no fertilisation has taken place, then the corpus luteum will degenerate and oestrogen and progesterone will decline, resulting in menstruation.
The **menstrual phase** lasts three to seven days and is where menses occur, at the end of which the endometrium will be 0.5 mm in thickness.

SEXUAL INTERCOURSE

Both men and women experience during sexual intercourse the sexual response cycle. This follows four phases: **desire, excitement, plateau, orgasm** and **resolution. Desire** is influenced through stimuli that can be from many different areas such as environmental and cultural, and causes the initiation or receptiveness of sexual activity. **Excitement** develops through stimulation. **Plateau** is a consolidation period in which intense stimulation will be intensified. **Orgasm** is where there are involuntary contractions causing the peaking of sexual pleasure and the release in sexual tension. **Resolution** is where the body returns to its pre-excitement state which can be seen in loss of erection or the decrease in the clitoris's size, and vasocongestion is relieved. If orgasm does not occur, then discomfort in the genital area may be experienced, as vasocongestion has not been relieved.

The sexual response cycle can be influenced by cultural, religious and personal experiences. Communication between sexual partners is a vital aspect of satisfying sexual intercourse; however, this is not always an area that people feel confident enough to discuss with their sexual partners and so can lead to loss of libido, or failure to achieve orgasm or premature ejaculation, for example. Psychosexual counselling of the individual or couple can address psychological causes and is available through referral in most sexual health services.

THE MALE

When a man is aroused, the penis becomes erect through the dilatation of arterioles in corpus spongiosum and corpora cavernosa, the erectile tissue inside the penis. The arterioles dilate and become engorged with blood; the penis becomes enlarged in length and width. An erection can occur through direct stimulation or from thought, visual or emotional material, and is controlled by spinal reflex. The erection reflex can begin with the stimulation of highly sensitive mechanoreceptors at the tip of the penis. The afferent synapse in the lower spinal cord and the efferent flow via the nervi erigentes produce the relaxation in the arterioles in the corpus spongiosum and corpora cavernosa. At the same time, parasympathetic nerves stimulate the urethral glands to produce a secretion to aid lubrication and entry of the erect penis into the vagina. Following ejaculation, men experience a refractory period in which they are unable to ejaculate further, although they may be capable of partial erection.

THE FEMALE

When a woman is sexually excited, the clitoris and the labia minora will become erect, the breasts will enlarge and the nipples will become erect. The vagina will become lubricated, and this will aid vaginal penetration by the penis. Women achieve orgasm through the stimulation of the clitoris and the cervix; they are able to achieve several orgasms within a short period of time. Orgasm causes the cervix and uterus to contract rhythmically, aiding the aspiration of sperm into the uterus. Orgasm is not necessary for fertilisation. Women do not experience a refractory period, so they may be able to experience repeated orgasms before experiencing resolution.

THE EFFECT OF AGE ON MEN AND WOMEN

Menopause usually occurs in women between the ages of 45 and 55; the mean age in the UK is 48 years. Menopause is the permanent cessation of menses with loss of ovarian function. It is defined as 12 months of no menstruation, which can only be diagnosed retrospectively. During menopause, there is a deficiency of oestrogen and progesterone. The hypothalamus responds by increasing gonadotrophins. FSH and LH can be ten times the normal menstruating woman's levels. The reduction of oestrogen and progesterone and increase of follicle-stimulating and luteinizing hormones result in menopausal symptoms. Menopausal symptoms can vary between women, but women can complain of vaginal dryness, hot flushes or headaches. Women under the age of 50 should use contraception for two years after their last menstrual period, and women over the age of 50 should be advised to use contraception for one year after their last period (FSRH, 2010).

From the age of 55 or older, men tend to have fewer firm erections, produce smaller amounts of semen and experience less intense ejaculations, with less need to ejaculate and a longer resolution period. Erectile dysfunction in men under the age of 40 is likely to be caused by psychological issues. However, in men over 40 who experience erectile dysfunction, this can be a warning sign of hidden medical problems such as diabetes, hypertension or raised cholesterol.

In two out of three men with hypertension, erectile dysfunction is experienced; just as the coronary arteries to the heart can be occluded with atheroma so can the arteries to the penis, causing problems with erections. Men should be encouraged to keep their weight and cholesterol within normal limits, not to smoke and keep fit not just for their hearts but also for a healthy sex life.

CASE STUDY 2.1

Joe is a 50-year-old man who attends a sexual health clinic complaining of problems whilst having sexual intercourse. On discussion, he admits he has problems getting an erection; he is not taking any other medications and has no medical history. On history taking, he admits that he smokes 20 cigarettes a day and drinks 30 units a week of alcohol. His height is 177 cm, and his weight is 95 kg. Body mass index (BMI) is 30.3. Blood pressure is 160/105. On discussion, Joe reveals that he does not get erections at all and no longer gets early morning erections. He is very worried about the situation.

Joe is a good example of the consequences of high blood pressure caused by smoking, alcohol and possibly high cholesterol. He will need to be referred for hypertensive treatment and be screened for cholesterol and liver function, urea and electrolytes.

As Joe is no longer getting early morning erections, this is unlikely to be a psychosexual issue and likely to be caused by atheroma reducing the blood flow to the penis. As a result, Joe needs to be referred to an erectile dysfunction clinic so that they can help him with this problem.

FURTHER READING

If you are interested in this area, then you may find the following websites useful.
Sexual Advice Association – www.sda.uk.net
British Society for Sexual Medicine – www.bssm.org.uk

4

FERTILITY AWARENESS

INTRODUCTION

Natural family planning methods have been used widely in the past by various religious groups, such as the Roman Catholic faith. They involve the observation of certain body changes which denote ovulation. From this information, a couple may choose to either abstain from sexual intercourse and use it as their family planning method or use this fertile period to have sexual intercourse promoting pregnancy, known as fertility awareness.

HISTORY OF THESE METHODS

Natural family planning methods have been referred to previously as periodic abstinence, the safe period and the rhythm method. It is only more recently that they have been promoted to women as a fertility awareness method, and as more women are delaying pregnancy, they have become a popular choice. Infertility clinics may ask women at initial consultations to use fertility awareness kits; previously, they used the temperature method to indicate ovulation.

In 1930, Ogino in Japan, and in 1933, Klaus in Austria, found that conception took place in-between menstrual cycles, and the time from ovulation to the next menstrual period was always the same regardless of the cycle. Using this information, they developed the calendar method. Around this period, changes in the cervical mucus were noted by Seguy and Vimeux. Ferin, in 1947, first noticed that a woman's body temperature changed at ovulation. However, it was not until 1964 that Drs John and Evelyn Billings used these discoveries to formulate the Billings method, now known as the cervical method.

Recently, research has increased in this area, there are now apps to help you monitor your temperature and record your cycle, and there is the persona contraception system, which uses urinary dipsticks to monitor oestrogen and luteinizing hormone in urine. The temperature method has benefitted from electronic and digital thermometers by increasing accuracy and decreasing the time clients need to take their temperature.

EXPLANATION OF THE METHOD

There are four main natural family planning and fertility awareness methods:

1. The temperature method.
2. The cervical mucus method (previously known as the Billings method).

DOI: 10.4324/9781003484424-5

3. The calendar method.
4. Combination of methods, also known as the sympto-thermal method or double-check method.

These methods help a woman to recognise when ovulation takes place. This usually occurs between days 12 and 16 before the next menstrual period. The ovum remains capable of being fertilised for 12–24 hours, whilst sperm are capable of fertilising the ovum for three to five days and on occasions have survived up to seven days *in utero* (see Figure 4.1).

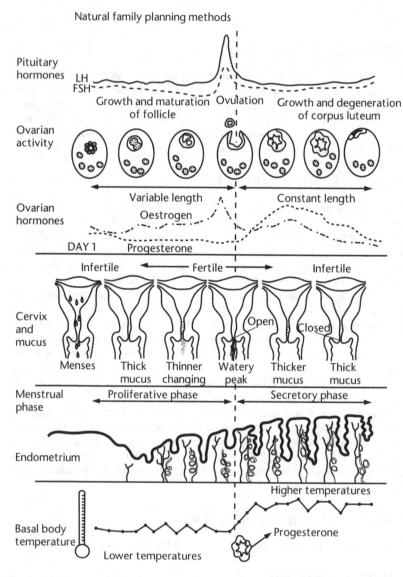

Figure 4.1 Changes during the menstrual cycle (reproduced with kind permission from E. Clubb & J. Knight, 1996).

During each menstrual cycle, the pituitary gland releases **follicle-stimulating hormone** (FSH). This triggers the development of follicles, which contain the immature ova, and is known as the **follicular phase**. As the follicles develop, they secrete the hormone oestrogen. This causes the reduction of FSH so that further ovum development is inhibited, the endometrium becomes thickened ready for implantation and the cervical glands produce mucus favourable to sperm penetration. As the ovum ripens, the level of oestrogen rises, causing the pituitary gland to produce **luteinizing hormone** (LH). This causes the follicle to rupture, releasing the ovum into the fallopian tube; this is known as **ovulation**. Rising oestrogen levels cause the cervix to soften and rise upwards and the os to open. The empty follicle becomes the **corpus luteum**, which secretes the hormone progesterone. This part of the menstrual cycle is known as the **luteal phase**. Progesterone causes the basal body temperature to rise during the luteal phase after ovulation. The pituitary gland is now inhibited from producing LH and FSH so that further ovulation is prevented. Following ovulation, cervical mucus becomes thickened and sticky, making sperm penetration difficult. The cervix becomes firm and the os closes. If the ovum is fertilised, then the corpus luteum will continue to produce progesterone throughout early pregnancy. However, if the ovum is not fertilised, then the corpus luteum will disintegrate, the level of progesterone will drop and menstruation will occur. The shift in basal body temperature, position of the cervix and change in cervical mucus are all used as indicators for natural family planning and fertility awareness to assess when a woman is fertile.

EFFICACY

The efficacy of natural family planning methods is 80%–98% with careful use. The sympto-thermal is the most effective method, as it uses a combination of methods. In theory, the efficacy of the sympto-thermal method can be as high as 98%; however, with this and any natural family planning method, the range of effectiveness of the method is dependent on the user and is known as the user failure rate. The efficacy is dependent on the level of motivation and commitment the couple gives to the method. Many men and women use this method to space their pregnancies, and as a result may be prepared to take more risks – a pregnancy slightly earlier than planned may be a happy accident! However, couples who are using the method to avoid pregnancy are more likely to be highly motivated and conscientious; they are less likely to take risks, so the user failure rate will be lower and the efficacy higher. Lastly, the level and expertise of the teaching of this method will influence the efficacy of the method, which is why it is vital that this method is taught by a teacher trained in natural family planning. If you are interested in training in natural methods or need to refer a client to a trainer, you should access the Fertility UK website (www.fertilityuk.org), which is an excellent source of information.

UKMEC

The UKMEC advises that there is limited evidence, but expert opinion advises that women who wish to use fertility awareness as contraception should stop hormonal contraception and have an established menstrual cycle (a minimum of three months) before relying on the fertility awareness as a method of contraception (FSRH, 2015a). It is also advised that women who are taking teratogenic drugs or who have a significant health risk avoid using fertility awareness as a method of contraception (FSRH, 2015a). This should be discussed with the woman and all medical teams involved so that a management plan can be formulated.

Disadvantages of natural family planning methods

- Requires motivation
- Needs to be taught by a specialist in natural family planning
- Requires the observation and recording of changes in the body
- May take time to learn and so may require a period of abstinence

Advantages of natural family planning methods

- Under the control of the couple once learnt
- Inexpensive (except in the personal contraceptive method)
- Can be used to promote pregnancy
- Increases couple's knowledge of changes in the body and fertility
- No physical side effects
- Acceptable to some religious beliefs and cultures

TEMPERATURE METHOD

The temperature method involves the woman taking her temperature every day to record her basal body temperature. Following ovulation, the basal body temperature (BBT) will drop slightly and then rise by 0.2°C–0.4°C where it will stay until the next period. This occurs because after ovulation, the hormone progesterone is secreted by the corpus luteum, which causes a woman's BBT to rise (see Figure 4.1).

The client should be advised to take her temperature at the same time each day before getting out of bed. If she works night shift, she should do this after sleeping in the evening. She should take her temperature first before drinking or eating, as these will affect the BBT. The thermometer should be an ovulation thermometer, which is calibrated in tenths of a degree between the range of 35°C and 39°C. A digital or electronic thermometer may be used, which takes about 45 seconds to give a reading. The temperature can be taken orally, which takes five minutes, or vaginally or rectally, which takes three minutes. The temperature should always be taken by the same route to avoid inaccuracy. The temperature is recorded on a chart commencing on the first day of her menstrual period (see Figure 4.2). Once the temperature has risen and has been maintained for three days, then the couple may have unprotected sexual intercourse until the first day of the next menstrual period (Figure 4.2).

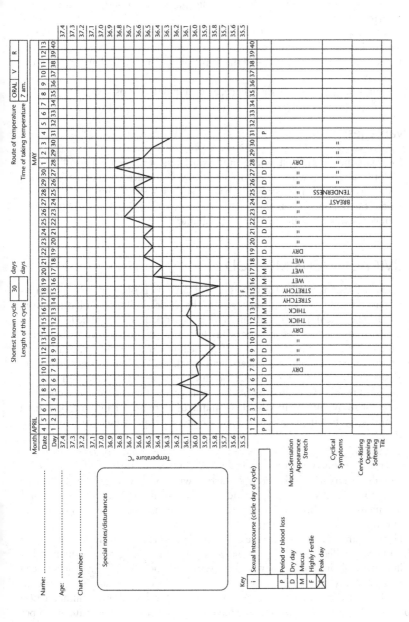

Figure 4.2 Temperature chart.

Disadvantages

- Requires motivation
- Needs to be taught by a specialist in natural family planning
- BBT is affected by illness, disturbed sleep, stress, alcohol and drugs, e.g. aspirin
- If the temperature is not taken at roughly the same time each day, this will lead to inaccuracies in the BBT
- Does not detect the beginning of the fertile period, making it harder to achieve pregnancy
- Requires long periods of abstinence, as it only detects post ovulation

Advantages

- Increases the couple's knowledge and awareness of the fertile period
- Helpful to women who experience erratic cycles by detecting ovulation
- Can help to pinpoint other body changes such as cervical mucus
- Under the woman's control
- Can be used to prevent or promote pregnancy

CERVICAL MUCUS METHOD

The cervical mucus method involves a woman observing her cervical mucus every day. The mucus varies throughout the cycle. Following menstruation, there is little cervical mucus, and this is often described as "dry." The level of the hormones oestrogen and progesterone are low, and the mucus is known as infertile mucus. There may be an absence of cervical mucus, or it may appear sticky, and, if stretched between two fingers, will break. As the ovum begins to ripen, increasing amounts of oestrogen are produced, causing an increase in cervical mucus. This marks the beginning of the fertile phase. Oestrogen levels continue to rise prior to ovulation, and the cervical mucus increases in amount, becoming clear and stretchy; if held between two fingers it can stretch easily without breaking.

It has been described as looking like raw egg white and is called fertile mucus. The last day of this type of mucus is known as peak mucus day, which can only be identified retrospectively. Four days following peak mucus day the mucus becomes thick, sticky and opaque, and is known as infertile mucus. This change in the mucus occurs because the ovum has been released and the level of oestrogen has dropped (see Figure 4.3).

The woman is taught to observe and record her cervical mucus several times a day either by collecting some on toilet paper or by inserting her fingers into her vagina to check its consistency and appearance. She will also be encouraged to become aware of changes in sensation of her cervical mucus. Trials (Indian Council of Medical Research Task Force on Natural Family Planning, 1996) looking at the cervical mucus method have shown a method failure rate of 1.5 per 100 users and a user failure rate of the method of 15.9 per 100 users at 21 months. This would seem to illustrate how vital training and motivation of the client and her partner are in ensuring efficacy.

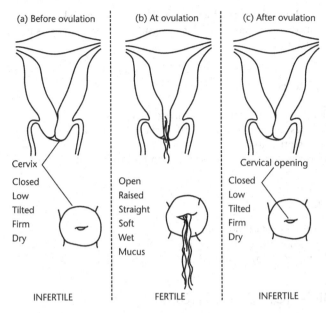

(a) Before ovulation

(b) At ovulation

(c) After ovulation

Cervix

Cervical opening

Closed	Open	Closed
Low	Raised	Low
Tilted	Straight	Tilted
Firm	Soft	Firm
Dry	Wet	Dry
	Mucus	

INFERTILE

FERTILE

INFERTILE

Figure 4.3 Changes in the cervix during the menstruation cycle (reproduced with kind permission from E. Clubb & J. Knight, 1996).

Disadvantages

- Requires commitment
- Needs to be taught by a specialist in natural family planning
- Can take two or three cycles to learn the method
- Vaginal infections can make it difficult to identify fertile mucus
- Some drugs used for treatment of colds, for example, can inhibit cervical mucus production
- Involves touching the body, which some women may dislike
- Requires abstinence

Advantages

- Under the control of the woman
- Gives the couple permission to touch their bodies
- Increases awareness of body changes
- Predicts fertile mucus, thus enabling pregnancy
- Can be used to prevent pregnancy

CALENDAR METHOD

The calendar method involves a woman detecting when her fertile period is, which is usually 12–16 days before the first day of her next menstrual period. This is based on looking retrospectively over the woman's menstrual cycle for a period of 6–12 months of recorded cycles. This method is no longer recognised as reliable on its own but may be taught alongside another method, as in the combination of methods.

Disadvantages

- Unreliable as it does not consider irregular cycles
- Stress, illness and travelling can affect the menstrual cycle
- Requires motivation
- Requires menstrual cycle to be recorded for 6–12 months prior to use

Advantages

- Under the control of the woman
- Increases knowledge about fertility
- Can be used in conjunction with another method

COMBINATION OF METHODS

This is often referred to as the sympto-thermal method or double-check method and combines the temperature, calendar and cervical mucus methods, which is why it is more effective as a contraceptive. Women are also encouraged to observe changes in their cervix such as consistency, position, and whether their cervical os is open or closed. During the beginning of the cycle when the levels of oestrogen and progesterone are reduced, the cervix is positioned low in the vagina and can be easily felt. The cervical os is closed, and the cervix feels firm to the touch. As oestrogen levels increase, the cervix changes and at peak mucus day feels soft. The os is now open, and the cervix has risen higher into the vagina, making it harder to locate. Following ovulation, the cervix returns to its former state, positioned lower, and feels firmer with the os closed. Checking the position and consistency of the cervix; along with the cervical mucus method, can easily be performed by either partner. Women are encouraged to observe and record mood changes and breast tenderness, which usually occur in the latter part of the cycle. They may be aware of ovulation pain (known as **mittelschmerz**) and/or mid-cycle bleeding. All these indicators help to confirm changes in the cycle.

Disadvantages

- Requires motivation
- Needs to be taught by a specialist in natural family planning
- Requires daily commitment

Advantages

- Detects beginning and end of fertile phase
- Can be used to promote pregnancy

■ Higher contraceptive efficacy than any other single natural family planning method

LACTATIONAL AMENORRHOEA METHOD

The lactational amenorrhoea method (LAM) is the use of breast feeding to inhibit ovulation and act as a contraceptive. If a woman has a baby of less than six months old and is amenorrhoeic and fully breast feeding, then there is only about a 2% chance of pregnancy occurring. However, if a woman is not fully breast feeding or not amenorrhoeic, then the risk of pregnancy will be greater. Many women will choose to rely upon another method of contraception such as barrier methods or the progestogen-only pill, as well as LAM.

One of the difficulties with this method is that women in the western world are encouraged and motivated to stop night-time feeding, and this may not give enough stimulation to inhibit ovulation.

Case history

A 51-year-old woman consulted having used natural family planning all her fertile life. She had used no other contraceptive method and had had three planned pregnancies. She was finding it difficult to identify when ovulation was occurring and was finding long periods of abstinence unsatisfactory.

Following discussion with the woman, she agreed that she and her partner would use condoms, and she would continue with natural family planning. She decided that a diaphragm would stop her being able to use the natural family planning method, as the use of a spermicide would affect the detecting of changes in the cervical mucus.

THE FUTURE

New innovations in natural family planning have focused on making the methods accessible to women. The standard days method uses the knowledge of fertility awareness methods to identify the fertile window of days 8–19 of the cycle and avoid unprotected sexual intercourse (Sinai et al., 2012). These methods are particularly useful in countries where contraception is limited, as seen in research undertaken in Ethiopia (Bekele, 2012). CycleBeads were used in Ethiopia to illustrate the standard days method; these are a string of beads which represent each day of the cycle; they are coloured white or brown, with white beads indicating days you can get pregnant and brown beads are days when you are not likely to get pregnant. The standard days method is advocated for women with cycles of 26–32 days. This method offers important solutions to women throughout the world, is inexpensive, easy to use and within the power of the woman.

SEXUALITY AND ANXIETIES

Women who choose natural family planning methods as a contraceptive or as a means of becoming pregnant can find this method empowering; it gives them control of their lives and gives them information about their bodies that is often concealed from them. As a method, it gives men and women permission to investigate and touch a woman's body. Sometimes when a woman tries this method, she finds that her cycle is not as regular as she first thought, leading to longer periods of abstinence than initially anticipated (Flynn, 1996). However, it may be argued that periodic abstinence can enhance a relationship, giving women and their partners time to enjoy a non-penetrative sexual relationship, creating greater understanding of each other (Ryder & Campbell, 1995).

For women who choose this method, it can be empowering; freedom of choice allows this. However, for some women, for moral or religious reasons, this is the only acceptable method; this can feel very limiting and unsatisfactory. If a woman has experienced unwanted or several pregnancies, there may be anxiety about becoming pregnant again in the future, and it may be a good time to discuss this method and whether another method may be more suitable.

If either member of the couple has anxieties with this method – perhaps a partner does not want another pregnancy, or if used as a means of promoting pregnancy, then a partner may feel a pressure to "perform" – this may manifest itself with sexual dysfunction. Some male clients who feel a pressure to "perform" may complain of loss of libido or erectile problems. Women who are anxious about becoming pregnant may complain of loss of libido and lack of sexual enjoyment. These problems may be very difficult for the client to discuss, but it is important that during the consultation you listen to the feelings in yourself that are evoked by the consultation, e.g. anger or sadness, as these will help you to try to understand how your client feels about the situation and whether they may wish to be referred for psychosexual counselling.

ANSWERS TO SELF-ASSESSMENT QUESTIONS

1 What sort of problems with the natural family planning method do you think your client may encounter?

Your client may encounter problems locating her cervix or may find it difficult to distinguish between the changes in the cervical mucus. She may find it difficult to remember to take her temperature every day at the same time, especially if she has young children or works shifts.

If she is unwell or has had a disturbed sleep pattern, then this will affect her BBT. Events like late-night parties, children waking in the night and alcohol consumption will all affect the BBT. If your client's cycle has been affected by a change in hormone levels and she has secondary amenorrhoea, for example following pregnancy or at menopause, she may find it difficult to interpret her fertile phase, and another method may be more appropriate.

2 How would you solve these problems?

If your client has difficulty locating her cervix, then she will need to be taught. She may find it easier to feel her cervix if she uses a squatting position or in a standing position with one foot on a chair and if she tries feeling in her infertile phase when the cervix is lower and easier to feel.

If there are problems distinguishing between the changes in the cervical mucus, then it is important to eliminate vaginal infection, which would camouflage normal discharge. Your client may lack confidence and knowledge in her mucus changes; it may be a good idea to book more frequent consultations so that you can check the cervical mucus together throughout her cycle.

Difficulty remembering temperature taking may be solved with an alarm. A digital thermometer may be useful, as it only takes 45 seconds to record the temperature, and if a mother is rushing out of bed for a crying child, this may be a suitable compromise. The problem may signify the woman's dissatisfaction with the method, and another method may be more suitable.

3 For whom do you think this method might be unsuitable and why?

Women who have a delay in ovulation caused by secondary amenorrhoea following childbirth or menopause would need to have long periods of abstinence, which makes this method unsuitable for these women.

Other women who would be considered unsuitable for this method are women who do not want to get pregnant and require a contraceptive with a high efficacy. The method would be unsuitable for women for whom pregnancy would be detrimental to their health or that of their foetuses, e.g. following administration of a live vaccine when teratogenesis is a risk.

4 Which day of a woman's menstrual cycle is counted as the first day?

The first day of a woman's menstrual cycle is counted as the first day of her period. Many women think that the first day of their cycle is at the end of their period.

5 If a woman has a regular menstrual cycle of 5/35 days, when is she most likely to be fertile?

A woman ovulates between 12 and 16 days before her next period; therefore, a woman with a regular 35-day cycle would be fertile between days 19 and 23 of her cycle.

6 If a woman has a regular menstrual cycle of 3/21 days, when is she most likely to be fertile?

A woman with a regular 21-day cycle would be fertile between days 5 and 8 of her cycle.

SEXUALLY TRANSMITTED INFECTIONS

5

INTRODUCTION

Sexual intercourse is a fundamental part of being human; with it arise risks such as pregnancy. Much of this book focuses on avoiding unwanted pregnancy; however, a huge risk of sexual intercourse is sexually transmitted infections. There are many views about sexually transmitted infections; many men and women believe that they are not at risk; others will see it as "par for the course" and others will be horrified. But whatever views they hold, STIs have a huge psychological and emotional impact alone without adding in the repercussions to fertility.

HISTORY

Syphilis was documented as early as the 15th century and was known as the great pox because of its long incubation period; it was not associated with sexual intercourse for some time. In the 18th century, it was known that syphilis and gonorrhoea were venereal diseases. During the First World War, when there was an increase in the incidence of syphilis and gonorrhoea, a Royal Commission on Venereal Diseases in 1916 set up a network of national clinics to help treat the problem. The second surge of STIs occurred following the Second World War, and in 1948, the National Health Service took over these clinics.

Today, clinics known as sexual health clinics are increasingly integrated with contraception to provide both services. Information in sexual health clinics is anonymised to maintain confidentiality and is not disclosed without clients' consent to general practitioners; every effort is made to ensure that patients' confidentiality is maintained to encourage men and women to attend.

TAKING A SEXUAL HISTORY

When commencing your consultation, you will want to discuss confidentiality; throughout your session, you will want to ascertain whether this is consenting sexual intercourse, whether the person is under 18 years and needs to be assessed for child safeguarding or whether they are a vulnerable adult, and adult safeguarding teams need to be involved. Your client may have been sexually assaulted, and you should be watching for anything that gives you concern that this has occurred so that you can tailor your care around this.

When taking a sexual history, it is important to find out what has brought the person to the clinic: Are they anxious about a particular episode of sexual

DOI: 10.4324/9781003484424-6

intercourse or a rash, for example? This will also help when you cover the issue of window periods for sexually transmitted infections, as the episode may/may not be covered, and they may have to repeat the screening.

You will also need to know if they are taking any other medications, their medical history and whether they are allergic to anything. If they are a woman, you will need to know when their last menstrual period was so you can eliminate pregnancy or perform a pregnancy test if indicated. You will also need to know what form of contraception the woman uses.

You then need to ask about whether they have symptoms; if they are asymptomatic, you can do an asymptomatic screen. If they have any of the symptoms listed in Table 5.1, they will need to be examined.

It is useful to find out how long they have had the symptoms and whether they have worsened. If they have pain, does the pain come and go, or is it there all the time? What makes the pain worse? If your client is a woman, you should consider performing a pregnancy test as this could be an ectopic pregnancy or pelvic inflammatory disease (PID).

Has your client had any sexually transmitted infections? When was this? Where were they treated? It is possible if this was recently that they may still have the infection, and you should consider treatment failure. This could be because of the following:

- **Poor compliance** – patients not completing antibiotic courses.
- **Reinfection** – patients not abstaining from sexual intercourse for seven days after completing treatment or having sexual intercourse with a partner who is still infected.
- **Antibiotic resistance** – most likely with gonorrhoea infections, which is why cultures are performed to ensure that an antibiotic is given which it is sensitive to.
- **Drug interaction/poor absorption** – the most likely cause is vomiting within two hours of ingesting azithromycin treatment for chlamydia, for example.

Table 5.1 Symptoms of male and female STIs

Symptoms for men	Symptoms for women
Discharge from penis	Discharge from vagina which is different from normal
Dysuria – pain or discomfort passing urine	Dysuria – pain or discomfort passing urine
Frequency of micturition	Frequency of micturition
Testicular pain	Abdominal pain
Rashes, lumps or sores in genital area	Rashes, lumps or sores in genital area
Discharge/bleeding from anus	Abnormal vaginal bleeding, postcoital bleeding
	Discharge/bleeding from anus
	Dyspareunia

You will also need to find out about your client's sexual partners for the last three months; this helps to clarify the risk of infection and the type of sexual intercourse to ensure correct screening. This is best achieved by asking when the client's last sexual intercourse was, was this a male or female partner, how long have they been having sexual intercourse, what type of sexual intercourse – oral, vaginal, anal –and did they use a condom? This could be abbreviated to the following:

LSI–2/7 cfp 3/12 vi – condom used, oi no condom

(Last sexual intercourse two days ago with casual female partner of three months, vaginal intercourse with a condom, oral intercourse, no condom used.)

You would next ask about the previous sexual partner for the next three months.

PSP 1–5/7 rfp 12/12 vi no condom used

(Previous sexual partner 1 – last sexual intercourse with them five days ago regular female partner of one year, vaginal intercourse, no condom used.)

PSP 2–1/12 cmp 1/7 oi r no condom. Ai i+r condom used

(Previous sexual partner 2 – last sexual intercourse with them one month ago with a casual male partner, one episode. Received oral sex, no condom used, insertive and receptive anal intercourse with a condom.)

This would tell you that this male client would need rectal, oral and urethral screening. You should discuss the risks of hepatitis A and B. Screening and immunisation for these should be completed if not done already. This is because anal sex has a higher risk, and he has sex with men.

It is important that you ask all clients and don't make assumptions about their sexuality, as this can lead to you missing someone who may be at risk. Finally, if a client requires a genital examination, you should have undergone training to do this; if you are not trained to do these procedures, you would need to refer the client to a sexual health clinic.

SCREENING FOR STIS IN ASYMPTOMATIC MEN AND WOMEN

Prior to performing any test, you should discuss what the test is for and any window period, the implications of a positive result and how the client will receive the results. Clients may choose not to screen for all STIs and may wish to have more time before considering a Human Immunodeficiency Virus (HIV) test, for example. It is important that clients have enough information so that they are able to consent.

If a man or a woman is asymptomatic, then they can be screened for chlamydia and gonorrhoea. A woman can do a vaginal self-swab; this is more sensitive in women than a urine test. A man can do a urine test and should not have passed urine for two hours. The most sensitive test for gonorrhoea and chlamydia available is a NAAT test (nucleic acid amplification test), and this will pick up infection from 14 days ago.

Blood tests for HIV and syphilis (serum treponemal serology – STS) should be discussed with all patients; a fourth-generation HIV test will give the result of HIV infection from four weeks ago. Fourth-generation HIV tests are the most sensitive form of testing for HIV antibodies and P24 antigens, and have a 99%–100% sensitivity. Third-generation HIV tests are still available but not first choice, as they are less accurate. You should be aware of the type of screening available in your area. Third-generation HIV tests have a window period of three months and so will give a result from three months prior to the test; they only screen for HIV antibodies, as these are detectable only after three months and 98.9% sensitive. HIV screening should be encouraged in all men and women, but those who are particularly at risk are those who come from geographical areas where HIV is widespread such as sub-Saharan Africa, men who have sex with men (MSM), intravenous drug users (IVDUs), commercial sex workers, victims of sexual assault, those with needle stick injuries and people who have an existing acute episode of an STI.

In early syphilis, the serology may be negative, so if this is suspected, the test should be repeated in three months. Hepatitis A IgG screening should be considered for MSM; if this does not show any immunity to the infection, then they should be vaccinated. Hepatitis B core antibody screening should be considered for MSM and IVDUs, as well as patients who grew up in a tropical country such as China or Africa. If this is positive, they will need to be referred to the Liver Unit, and partners will need screening; if this is negative, then vaccination should be considered. Hepatitis B surface antibody is performed when previous vaccination has been done to detect the level of immunity and should be done every five years. Hepatitis C screening should be considered for IVDU and MSM who are HIV positive. If serology is positive, then the client will need to be referred to the Liver Unit; there is no vaccination for hepatitis C.

SCREENING FOR STIS IN SYMPTOMATIC MEN AND WOMEN

If a person is symptomatic, then they will need to be screened and examined. They may be expecting this, but it is important before you start that you explain what you are about to do and why you need to do it. You will need to discuss what tests you are considering doing and why, and what this will mean if they are positive to ensure that consent is gained. It is easy to forget the impact of a positive test on a relationship; however, it is important that clients agree to this and understand how and when they will get the results.

You should always offer a chaperone, whether the client is male or female, and ensure sufficient privacy is given during the examination.

SYMPTOMATIC WOMAN

For a symptomatic woman, you will perform a pregnancy test if she has any abdominal pain or had a late or abnormal period prior to examination; if positive, she will need to be seen by a doctor. A pregnancy test will give you a result from three weeks ago. If your client has any urinary symptoms, then you will need to perform a urinalysis and may want to send an MSU (midstream urine) to microbiology. If the pregnancy test is negative, and she is not complaining of abdominal pain, you will need to perform a speculum examination and take swabs for microbiology from the vagina and endocervix for gonorrhoea sensitivities, and a gonorrhoea and chlamydia NAAT from the endocervix. When performing a speculum examination, it is good practice not to use any lubricating gel, as this can obscure the sample; wetting the speculum with some warm water should be sufficient. If you are working in a sexual health clinic where microscopy is available, then a dry and wet slide will be done; the wet slide for trichomonas and dry slide will have samples from the urethra, cervix and vagina; once stained, it enables staff to diagnose bacterial vaginosis, candida and gonorrhoea. This helps to aid diagnosis and treatment.

If trained a bimanual examination should be performed to eliminate PID. All the time you should be observing whether the vulva, vagina and cervix look normal; you are looking for anything abnormal.

Blood tests for HIV, syphilis and hepatitis, if required, should be done. If a woman has an ulcer in the genital area, it could be genital herpes and a swab from this should be taken; it could also be syphilis, so serology is important to exclude this.

SYMPTOMATIC MAN

For a symptomatic man, you will need to examine him; this will include palpation of testes for lumps, checking the groin for raised lymph nodes (normally you should be unable to feel these); this could indicate a viral infection. You should observe the penis – does it look normal? Is he circumcised or not? If he has a foreskin, can the client move this easily so you can take a specimen from the urethra? If he has problems retracting his foreskin, then this should be taken seriously, and he will need to be seen by a doctor and may need to be referred to Accident and Emergency. If a man has discharge from his penis, then a urethral specimen should be taken for gonorrhoea sensitivities and, if microscopy is available, a dry slide; this should then be followed by a urine specimen for chlamydia and gonorrhoea NAAT, which should be the first voided urine sample, and urinalysis and MSU if urinary symptoms to exclude a urinary tract infection.

Blood tests for HIV, syphilis and hepatitis, if required, should be done. If a man has an ulcer in the genital area, it could be genital herpes, and a swab from this should be taken; it could also be syphilis, so serology is important to exclude this.

TYPES OF SEXUALLY TRANSMITTED INFECTIONS

Gonorrhoea

Neisseria gonorrhoea is caused by gram-negative diplococcus. It can be found in the urethra, endocervix, rectum, oropharynx and conjunctiva. In asymptomatic men and women where a NAAT test for gonorrhoea and chlamydia test have been found to be positive, a culture for gonorrhoea sensitivities needs to be performed to ensure the correct treatment is given. Men who are symptomatic with gonorrhoea have a muco-purulent urethral discharge which can be very profuse; they can have dysuria and pain and swelling of their testicles. Symptomatic women may present with discharge and abdominal pain. Pharyngeal infection is asymptomatic in 90% of men and women. Rectal infection is usually asymptomatic but may cause pain and discharge. This highlights why it is important to ask about the type of sexual intercourse clients have so you can screen the relevant area.

Treatment

First-line treatment recommended by the British Association for Sexual Health and HIV if not allergic to penicillin is ceftriaxone 1 g stat intramuscularly (Fifer et al., 2019).

All sexual partners for the last three months will need to be contacted for screening and treatment. Clients should be advised to have no sexual intercourse for one week, and they should return for a test of cure at two weeks.

Increasingly, gonorrhoea is becoming resistant to treatment, which is why a test of cure is so important. Currently, there is a phase 3 study of oral zoliflodacin being carried out to investigate alternative treatment for gonorrhoea (GARDP, 2023). An important resource is the gonococcal resistance to antimicrobials surveillance programme (GRASP) which provides up to date information on resistance and treatment of gonorrhoea and can be found at https://www.gov.uk/government/publications/gonococcal-resistance-to-antimicrobials-surveillance-programme-grasp-report.

Chlamydia

Chlamydia is a common infection which is usually asymptomatic. Complications include PID, ectopic pregnancy, infertility caused by fallopian tube damage in women and in men, it can cause prostatitis, epididymo-orchitis. Women may complain of dysuria, postcoital bleeding, irregular bleeding, deep dyspareunia or abdominal pain. Men may complain of clear urethral discharge, urethral irritation or dysuria. Pharyngeal infection is usually asymptomatic, and rectal infection can also be asymptomatic but may also cause pain and discharge. A diagnosis of gonorrhoea and chlamydia is made from a NAAT swab or can be done on a dry slide if microscopy is available and there are five or more pus cells.

Treatment

1 Doxycycline 100 mg bd for seven days (contraindicated in pregnancy)
2 Azithromycin 1g orally as a single dose, followed by 500 mg once daily for two days

Clients should be advised if they vomit within two hours, they will need to repeat the dose, and they should have no sexual intercourse for seven days, and all sexual partners for the last three months should be contacted.

Trichomoniasis

Trichomonas vaginalis is found in the urethra, paraurethral glands and vagina; it is caused by a flagellated protozoan and is sexually transmitted. It can be asymptomatic in men and women but can cause increased yellow frothy vaginal discharge, itching and dysuria in women, and in men, it can cause urethral discharge and dysuria. Diagnosis is with a wet slide and microscopy, or by specialist culture testing through a NAAT self-taken vaginal swab or first-void stream urine sample; however, this is still not widely available. Microscopy screening is more accurate for women and can be 80% sensitive, but it is difficult to diagnose in men and can have only a 30% sensitivity. Treatment first line is metronidazole 400 mg twice daily for five days; clients should be advised to not have sexual intercourse for seven days after treatment has been completed, and all sexual contacts for the previous three months should be treated.

Syphilis

Syphilis is caused by the bacteria *Treponema pallidum* and can be transmitted horizontally through sexual or blood borne infection or vertically through the placenta as congenital syphilis. It is classified as follows:

- Early syphilis is defined as the first two years of infection.
  1 Primary – this is early syphilis within the first 90 days of infection associated with a primary lesion known as a chancre; this is painless and looks like an ulcer. The ulcer is oval or round and has a clearly defined outline.
  2 Secondary – 6–12 weeks from infection, often associated with a symmetrical rash which can be found on the trunk and limbs, face, palms of the hands and soles of the feet.
- Early latent – defined as infection less than two years and asymptomatic.
- Late latent – defined as infection more than two years and asymptomatic.
- Tertiary or symptomatic late syphilis – untreated syphilis, which can involve the musculoskeletal, neurological and cardiovascular systems, which can result in aortic aneurysm, aortic regurgitation, paralysis, memory loss, antisocial behaviour and gumma formation (syphilitic granulation tissue).

Treatment

First-line treatment is benzathine penicillin 2.4 MU given intramuscularly two doses a week apart in early syphilis: in late syphilis three doses given weekly for three weeks. Clients with late syphilis should be examined to exclude any cardiac or neurological involvement. All men and women with syphilis should be advised not to have sexual intercourse until it is confirmed that they are not infectious. In early syphilis, all sexual partners in the last three months will need to be traced; if it is secondary or early latent syphilis, sexual contacts for the last two years will need to be informed. Clients will require regular serology to ensure that they have been successfully treated and there is no relapse.

Genital warts

Genital warts are mostly benign and are caused by the human papillomavirus types 6 and 11. Men and women find them embarrassing and distressing. They are diagnosed through visual inspection. Treatment for external genital warts is through cryotherapy followed by podophyllotoxin solution 0.5% treatment (if it is easy for the client to apply treatment to the wart); one week later, this is applied twice a day for three days per week for four weeks. Treatment should be applied only to broken skin, and warts should be reviewed in five weeks. Podophyllotoxin is contraindicated in pregnancy. Warts on the cervix will need referral to colposcopy. Treatment can cause scarring, and men and women should be advised to use condoms.

Genital herpes

Genital herpes is caused by the herpes simplex virus (HSV) types 1 and 2. HSV type 1 is associated with orolabial mucosa, and HSV type 2 is associated with sexually transmitted genital herpes. Men and women may complain of ulceration in the genital area, which would have started as a blister and been itchy or stinging. Depending on the location of the ulcer, this may cause problems with passing urine and may cause retention of micturition and phimosis in men. Clients may have felt generally unwell and tired beforehand. Diagnosis is through an HSV swab taken from the ulcer. Treatment – Aciclovir 200 mg orally five times a day for five days. The use of condoms is important to reduce transmission. Genital herpes has no permanent cure; clients may never get another episode or may get frequent episodes. Clients can be very distressed; they can feel betrayed that a partner has not told them of an infection and find it difficult to discuss their diagnosis with partners.

HUMAN IMMUNODEFICIENCY VIRUS (HIV)

There are two types of HIV: HIV 1 and HIV 2. HIV 1 is found worldwide, and HIV 2 is found in West Africa, Portugal, France, India and South America. HIV stands for Human Immunodeficiency Virus, and if left untreated leads to AIDS (Acquired Immunodeficiency Disease). HIV is contracted through vaginal, anal or oral sexual intercourse; through sharing needles; through infected blood products; and from mother to child during pregnancy.

The HIV virus attacks a type of white blood cell called the CD4 cell. So, when a person is HIV positive their CD4 count is monitored along with their viral load. The CD4 count will tell us how the illness is progressing. A high CD4 count shows a robust immune system, a low CD4 count will mean that the person will be vulnerable to infections. The viral load shows how much HIV virus there is, a low or undetectable viral load means someone is less infectious. If an HIV positive patient is taking antiretroviral medication, and they are taking it correctly, then they are likely to have an undetectable viral load. However, this does not mean they are cured; this means that the HIV virus is controlled, and they are less infectious.

The PARTNER study (2019) has shown that transmission of HIV positive partners taking antiretroviral therapy (ART) when their HIV viral load is suppressed is effectively zero to their partners. This has led to the message that U=U (undetectable equals untransmittable) campaign and shows how important it is to adhere to treatment.

The number of new HIV diagnoses among gay and bisexual men fell by 42% from 1,239 to 724 between 2019 and 2022 (UKHSA. 2023). However, HIV diagnoses are increasing in heterosexual men and women, particularly women, emphasising the importance of discussing safer sex and screening (UKHSA, 2023).

Treatment of HIV

The primary aim of treatment is to suppress the virus and reduce HIV related infections and diseases and reduce transmission. Treatment of HIV is with Antiretroviral Therapy (ART) which has improved, with reduced side effects.

Table 5.2 Progression of HIV if left untreated

- **Seroconversion**
- This may be a mild flu-like infection or more severe infection.
- This is the most infectious stage of the illness.
- **Asymptomatic stage of HIV**
- The individual may feel well with no symptoms.
- **Symptomatic HIV**
- The longer the person is without treatment, the more likely they will become symptomatic. Their immune system will be compromised and will be unable to fight infections or diseases.
- **Late stage of HIV**
- The person may become ill with cancer-related illnesses and other infections. These are known as AIDS-defining illnesses.
- **AIDS-defining illnesses**
- These include cancer, tuberculosis, pneumonia.
- These days, most people do not get to this stage because of drug treatment.

Usually, treatment is commenced with Tenofovir-AF and emtricitabine. However, there are lots of treatment options, and ART medication groups include the following:

- Nucleoside/nucleotide reverse transcriptase inhibitors (NRTIs), e.g. tenofovir disoproxil fumarate, tenofovir alafenamide, lamivudine, emtricitabine, abacavir, zidovudine
- Non-nucleoside reverse transcriptase inhibitors (NNRTIs), e.g. efavirenz, nevirapine, etravirine, doravirine, rilpivirine
- Boosted protease inhibitors (boosted PIs), e.g. atazanavir/ritonavir, lopinavir/ritonavir, darunavir/ritonavir, atazanavir/cobicistat, darunavir/cobicistat
- Integrase strand transfer inhibitors (INSTIs), e.g. raltegravir, dolutegravir, bictegravir, cabotegravir
- Boosted integrase strand transfer inhibitors (boosted INSTIs), e.g. elvitegravir
- C-C chemokine receptor 5 (CCR5) antagonists. Examples include maraviroc
- Fusion inhibitors, e.g. enfuvirtide
- Attachment inhibitors, e.g. fostemsavir
- Post-attachment inhibitors, e.g. ibalizumab
- Pharmacokinetic enhancers. Examples include ritonavir, cobicistat

ART and contraception

Antiretroviral Therapy medication may reduce the efficacy of hormonal contraception if they are an enzyme inducing drug (FSRH, 2023b). If the ART drug reduces hormonal contraception efficacy, this will affect combined hormonal methods, progestogen only pills, the progestogen implant and hormonal emergency contraception. The contraceptive effectiveness of the depot medroxyprogesterone acetate (DMPA) injectable, the levonorgestrel-releasing intrauterine device (LNG-IUD) and the copper intrauterine device (Cu-IUD) are not reduced with ART (FSRH, 2023b). Women should continue to use barrier contraception to reduce their risk of STIs.

ART medications can be checked for drug interactions via the website for University of Liverpool HIV drug interaction checker at https://www.hiv-druginteractions.org/ and the British HIV Association (BHIVA) provides guidelines on antiretroviral treatment for adults living with HIV-1 at www.bhiva.org.

Hepatitis

Hepatitis is the term used to describe inflammation of the liver caused by a virus or by damage to the liver. There are six types of hepatitis A, B, C, D, E and G. In sexual health, patients are screened for hepatitis B risks so that vulnerable individuals can be vaccinated. Hepatitis B is contracted through having vaginal, anal or oral sex without using a condom or dam; injecting drugs users sharing needles; needle stick injuries, having a tattoo or piercing with unsterilised equipment; through an infected blood transfusion; from mother to baby. Individuals vulnerable to hepatitis B should be screened and, if needed, vaccinated.

CASE HISTORY

Mark is a 50-year-old man. He is married with two children; he attends the sexual health clinic complaining of discharge from his penis. He says that he has had one sexual partner – his female wife of 20 years – and has had no other partners in that time. Mark is a reluctant historian, and you feel that Mark is not telling you everything.

On examination, he has a clear discharge from his penis, and an irritation inside his penis. Under the microscope, he is found to have non-specific urethritis which you treat with doxycycline. As non-specific urethritis (NSU) can be caused by bacterial infections in older men, you warn him that this may be the cause, but it may also be caused by chlamydia, which is sexually transmitted. You advise Mark to have no sexual intercourse whilst treated and for seven days afterwards. You encourage him to talk to his wife and encourage her to get screened. The NAAT test returns positive for chlamydia and blood tests for syphilis and HIV are performed and the results return syphilis positive and HIV negative.

Mark returns for treatment for syphilis. On further questioning, he tells you that he has had three male sexual partners in the last year. Because Mark is reluctant to divulge that he has sex with men, he has not been vaccinated against hepatitis, and his knowledge on safe sex is poor.

To ensure Mark is safer, you treat the syphilis with penicillin, and screen for hepatitis. You ask the health advisor to see him and educate him on his risks and discuss screening his wife and assess whether he will need further HIV tests.

NON-SEXUALLY TRANSMITTED INFECTIONS

Bacterial vaginosis

Bacterial vaginosis (BV) is not a sexually transmitted infection and is caused by an overgrowth of anaerobic organisms in the vagina. It causes a fishy-smelling vaginal discharge, with soreness and itching; it is associated in pregnancy with premature rupture of membranes, preterm birth and post-partum endometritis. Treatment first line is metronidazole 400 mg twice daily for five days; contact screening is not required. If a woman suffers from recurrent BV, you may wish to refer her to a specialist clinic, as she may have trichomonas, and her partner should be treated. Women should be encouraged to avoid washing the vagina with bath and beauty products. The vagina is a self-cleaning organ; these products clean out the natural flora in the vagina, causing an overgrowth of anaerobic organisms and BV. Woman often wash more often after sexual intercourse, so you will need to discuss how BV is caused to reduce recurrences.

Candida

Candida is caused by *Candida albicans* and is not sexually transmitted. It causes vulval itching and soreness; the discharge is white and thick like "cottage cheese." Diagnosis is through a vaginal swab for microbiology or through microscopy. Treatment first line is clotrimazole 500 mg pessary per vagina or fluconazole 150 mg if not pregnant, 150 mg stat orally. It is good practice to perform urinalysis to exclude diabetes mellitus and a full STI screen. You should also warn your client that treatment for candida may cause condoms to break.

SELF-ASSESSMENT QUESTIONS

Answers and discussion at the end of the chapter.

1   You are giving azithromycin for chlamydial infection; what other advice do you need to give?
2   When should you perform a test of cure for gonorrhoea infection?
3   Why is it better to know you are HIV positive?

CASE HISTORY

A 32-year-old woman attends, as she wants to be screened for sexually transmitted infections. She is asymptomatic and always uses condoms for vaginal sex. She has had three partners in the last three months and has oral and vaginal sex. She never uses condoms for oral sex. She performs a NAAT self-swab for chlamydia and gonorrhoea, and it is suggested that she has oral NAAT swabs for chlamydia and gonorrhoea and culture swabs for gonorrhoea sensitivities. She also has blood taken for HIV and STS.

She returns two weeks later after receiving a phone call, as she has a positive gonorrhoea result. She is quite shocked, as she had no idea you could get gonorrhoea in the mouth.

SEXUALITY AND ANXIETIES

Sexually transmitted infections can cause a huge amount of anxiety in men and women. Whilst men and women know about HIV, they often think it won't happen to them, so they put themselves at risk. With increasing STIs being reported, it is easy to say that people are taking more risks, but actually, a large proportion of this is because of increasing sensitivity of diagnostic tests, and the increasing numbers taking up testing. Health professionals need to discuss with men and women how to negotiate screening with their partners and condom use. We also need to be open minded about sexual practices so that men and women are able to talk about the risks they take and so we can address these.

Clients often do not realise the intimate nature of the questions we need to ask and can feel very embarrassed; this is one reason why you should see them on their own, as they are more likely to be honest without the presence of friends or partners.

Certain STIs such as genital herpes and HIV will have long-term repercussions to a person's sexual life; they may feel unclean, a danger to sexual partners. Many feel that they have been foolish in trusting a partner who has not divulged an infection; they feel angry and betrayed. As result they may require psychosexual counselling, or counselling from a health advisor to adjust to their diagnosis.

ANSWERS TO SELF-ASSESSMENT QUESTIONS

1 When you give azithromycin for treatment for chlamydial you should advise men and women to return if they vomit within two hours of taking it. They should not have sexual intercourse for seven days and not have sexual intercourse with partners until they are screened and treated, and seven days after treatment has been completed.

2 Test of cures for gonorrhoea should be performed at two weeks to ensure clients have been treated successfully.

3 It is a good idea to know if you are HIV positive because there is HIV 1 and HIV 2. HIV 1 is more virulent than HIV 2, and HIV 2 is resistant to NNRTIs, so if you are HIV 1 positive, you will have more treatment options and can protect yourself from contracting HIV 2. With treatment, your viral load will be low, which will mean you will be less infectious, and progression of the infection can be monitored.

COMBINED METHODS

6

INTRODUCTION

This chapter includes efficacy of contraceptive pills; the pharmacokinetics and pharmacodynamics; United Kingdom Medical Eligibility Criteria (UKMEC) categories; second- and third-generation combined methods; risks of combined methods; types of combined pills, disadvantages and advantages; tailored prescribing; how to use the method; loss of efficacy and drug interaction; problems encountered with the method; and what to cover in the consultation.

THE COMBINED CONTRACEPTIVE PILL

Introduction and history

The combined pill is today one of the most widely used methods of contraception; it is effective in reducing dysmenorrhoea and can be taken easily, stopped and started by the woman.

Explanation of the method

The combined oral contraceptive pill contains the hormones oestrogen and progestogen. The synthetic forms of these found in combined contraceptive methods are ethinylestradiol and progestogens in the form of gestodene, desogestrel, drospirenone, levonorgestrel and norethisterone.

It prevents pregnancy by

- inhibiting ovulation,
- making the endometrium unfavourable for implantation, and
- making the cervical mucus impenetrable to sperm.

Efficacy

The efficacy for the combined pill is over 99% with careful and consistent use; however, with less careful use it can be 91% (FSRH, 2019a, amended October 2023).

DOI: 10.4324/9781003484424-7

Pharmacokinetics and pharmacodynamics

It is important to understand how the combined oral contraceptive is metabolised when taken orally, as there are many potential interactions which can reduce the effectiveness of the combined oral contraception (COC) and could result in loss of contraception and pregnancy. Oral ethinylestradiols and progestogens found in the COC are absorbed in the small intestine and metabolised in the liver and excreted in urine and faeces. There is no enterohepatic recirculation of progestogens, so efficacy is unchanged by changes to gut flora (FSRH, 2019a, amended October 2023). However, ethinylestradiol is subject to enterohepatic recirculation, and this may vary from person to person and is believed to be important in contraceptive effectiveness (FSRH, 2019a, amended October 2023).

In the liver, ethinylestradiol and progestogens are subject to phase 1 and 11 cytochrome P450 enzymes, are conjugated to form glucuronides and sulphates and excreted via bile into the small intestine. The combined pill conjugates of ethinylestradiols are cleaved by intestine colonic bacteria, and the active ethinylestradiol is reabsorbed via enterohepatic circulation; this is known as "first pass metabolism." The absorption of ethinylestradiol and progestogens will be affected and efficacy reduced by severe diarrhoea and vomiting, and they may be affected by chelating drugs and drugs that alter gastric pH (FSRH, 2022b). As a result of the first pass metabolism, the efficacy of the COC may be affected by certain drugs, these are known as enzyme-inducing drugs which induce cytochrome P450 enzymes (seen in Table 6.8) increasing the metabolism of oestrogen and progestogen, and as a result reducing the efficacy of the COC.

New research has found that in a study of 350 women, 5% had a gene called CYP3A7*1C enzyme. CYP3A*1C is usually active in foetuses and then switched off at birth. CYPSA7*1C has been found to break down hormonal contraception and may affect contraceptive efficacy. Further research is needed to help understand the implications (Lazorwitz et al., 2019).

Disadvantages

- Needs to be taken regularly, carefully and consistently
- No protection against STIs and HIV
- Increased risk of circulatory disorders, such as hypertension, arterial disease and venous thromboembolism
- Increased risk of liver adenoma, cholestatic jaundice and gallstones
- Effect of COC on breast cancer (see p. 69)
- Unsuitable for smokers over the age of 35

Advantages

- Reliable and easily reversible
- Relief of dysmenorrhoea and menorrhagia
- Reduces risk of anaemia
- Reduces the risk of benign breast disease
- Relief of pre-menstrual symptoms
- Fewer ectopic pregnancies

- Reduction of ovarian cysts
- Less pelvic inflammatory disease
- Protects against endometrial and ovarian cancer

UKMEC 4 unacceptable health risk – absolute contraindications

- Pregnancy
- Breast feeding
- Less than six weeks post-partum
- Undiagnosed vaginal or uterine bleeding
- Past or present venous thrombosis
- Past or present arterial thrombosis
- Cardiovascular and ischaemic heart disease
- Complicated pulmonary hypertension, atrial fibrillation and subacute bacterial endocarditis
- Cardiomyopathy with impaired cardiac function
- Migraine with aura
- Cerebrovascular accident and transient ischaemic attacks
- Active disease of the liver, e.g. malignancy, hepatocellular adenoma, history of cholestatic jaundice, impaired liver function tests, acute viral hepatitis, severe compensated cirrhosis
- Current breast cancer
- Positive antiphospholipid antibodies
- Raynaud's disease with lupus anticoagulant – if present, this will increase coagulation
- Stevens–Johnson syndrome
- Acute pancreatitis
- Known thrombogenic mutations such as factor V Leiden, prothrombin mutation, protein S and protein C and antithrombin deficiencies
- Smokers over the age of 35
- Hypertension with a systolic of 160 mmHg or diastolic over 100 mmHg
- Prolonged immobility

UKMEC 3 risks outweigh the benefits of using method – relative contraindications

- Obesity (BMI over 35 kg m^2)
- Lipid disorders and diseases where high-density lipoprotein (HDL) is reduced, e.g. diabetes, hypertension
- Migraine without aura
- History of migraine with aura, which was more than five years ago, at any age
- History of migraine with aura more than five years ago
- Multiple risk factors for cardiovascular disease
- Hypertension with a systolic over 140–159 mmHg or diastolic over 90–99 mmHg
- Severe diabetes mellitus with complications such as retinopathy, neuropathy, vascular disease
- Carriers of known gene mutations linked to breast cancer BRCAS 1/BRCAS 2

- Past history of breast cancer initiation needs to be in discussion with oncology team
- History of cholestasis with a combined method
- Current and medically treated gallbladder disease
- Diseases whose drug treatment affects the efficacy of the combined pill, e.g. tuberculosis, epilepsy
- Complicated organ transplant
- Family history of arterial or venous disease in a first-degree relative below the age of 45
- Immobility

RANGE OF METHOD

Drug manufacturers have produced a wide range of combined pills (Table 6.1). There are two types of combined pills:

- Monophasic pills
- Triphasic pills

Commonly used combined pills are second- and third-generation pills. Second-generation pills contain progestogens called levonorgestrel and norgestimate, whilst third-generation combined pills contain desogestrel, gestodene and drospirenone.

Monophasic pills

The most widely used combined pill is a monophasic pill, which means that it contains the same amount of oestrogen and progestogen throughout its 21 days of pills, e.g. Gedarel 150/20, Akizza, Ambelina, Bimizza, Elevin, Mercilon, Femodette, Millinette 20/75, Sunya, Gedarel 150/30, Marvelon, Alenova, Munalea 150/30, Cimizt, Yasmin, Femodene, Katya, Maexeni, Levest, Microgynon 30, Ovranette, Rigevidon, Brevinor, Norimin and Norinyl-1.

Of these, six are 20 microgram pills: Mercilon, Millinette 20/75, Gederal 20/150, Femodette, Sunya 20/75 and Bimizza.

Triphasic pills

These are 21-day pills which contain varying amounts of oestrogen (usually two different levels) throughout the packet but have three different levels of progestogen in them, which are colour-coded, e.g. Synphase, Qlaira (Table 6.2).

ED pills

There is currently only one every day (ED) pill. Zoely 24-day monophasic pill with 4 inactive pills (Tables 6.3 and 6.4).

Combined methods

Table 6.1 Combined contraceptive pills

Combined pill name	Preparation	Manufacturer	Micrograms of oestrogen per pill	Micrograms of progestogen per pill	Type of progestogen
Gedarel 150/20	21-day monophasic pill	Consilient	20 mcg	150 mcg	Desogestrel
Bimizza	21-day monophasic pill	Morningside healthcare Ltd.	20 mcg	150 mcg	Desogestrel
Mercilon	21-day monophasic pill	Organon	20 mcg	150 mcg	Desogestrel
Akizza	21-day monophasic pill	Morningside Healthcare Ltd	20 mcg	75 mcg	Gestodene
Femodette	21-day monophasic pill	Bayer Schering	20 mcg	75 mcg	Gestodene
Millinette 20/75	21-day monophasic pill	Consilient	20 mcg	75 mcg	Gestodene
Sunya	21-day monophasic pill	Stragen	20 mcg	75 mcg	Gestodene
Gedarel 150/30	21-day monophasic pill	Consilient	30 mcg	150 mcg	Desogestrel
Marvelon	21-day monophasic pill	Organon	30 mcg	150 mcg	Desogestrel
Akizza	21-day monophasic pill	Morningside Healthcare Ltd	30 mcg	75 mcg	Gestodene
Cimizt	21-day monophasic pill	Mornings-de Healthcare	30 mcg	150 mcg	Desogestrel
Yasmin	21-day monophasic pill	Bayer Schering	30 mcg	3 mg	Drospirenone
Femodene	21-day monophasic pill	Bayer Schering	30 mcg	75 mcg	Gestodene
Katya	21-day monophasic pill	Stragen	30 mcg	75 mcg	Gestodene
Millinette 30/75	21-day monophasic pill	Consilient	30 mcg	75 mcg	Gestodene
Levest	21-day monophasic pill	Mornings-de Healthcare	30 mcg	150 mcg	Levonorgestrel
Microgynon 30	21-day monophasic pill	Bayer	30 mcg	150 mcg	Levonorgestrel
Ambellina	21-day monophasic pill	Crescent Pharma Ltd	30 mcg	150 mcg	Levonorgestrel
Elevin	21-day monophasic pill	Mornings-de Healthcare	30 mcg	150 mcg	Levonorgestrel
Maexeni	21-day monophasic pill	Lupin Healthcare Ltd	30 mcg	150 mcg	Levonorgestrel
Ovranette	21-day monophasic pill	Pfizer	30 mcg	150 mcg	Levonorgestrel
Rigevidon	21-day monophasic pill	Consilient	30 mcg	150 mcg	Levonorgestrel
Brevinor	21-day monophasic pill	Pharmacia	35 mcg	500 mcg	Norethisterone
Norimin	21-day monophasic pill	Pharmacia	35 mcg	1 mg	Norethisterone
Norinyl-1	21-day monophasic pill	Pharmacia	Mestranol 50 mcg	1 mg	Norethisterone

Table 6.2 Phasic combined contraceptive pills

Combined pill name	Preparation	Manufacturer	Micrograms of oestrogen per pill	Micrograms of progestogen per pill	Type of progestogen
Synphase	7 pills 9 pills 5 pills	Pharmacia	35 mcg	500 mcg 1 mg 500 mcg	Norethisterone-one

Table 6.3 Combined ED contraceptive pills

Combined pill name	Preparation	Manufacturer	Micrograms of oestrogen per pill	Micrograms of progestogen per pill	Type of progestogen
Zoely	24-day monophasic pill with 4 inactive pills	Bayer PLC	1.5 mg oestradiol	2.5 mg	Nomegestrol acetate

Table 6.4 Combined phasic ED contraceptive pills

Combined pill name	Preparation	Number of pills per cycle	Manufacturer	Micrograms of oestrogen per pill	Micrograms of progestogen per pill	Type of progestogen
Qlaira	26-day pill with 2 inactive pills	2 pills 5 pills 17 pills 2 pills 2 inactive	Bayer Schering	Estradiol valerate 3 mg Estradiol valerate 2 mg Estradiol valerate 2 mg Estradiol valerate 1 mg	2 mg 3 mg	Dienogest

Tailored regimens

Taking the combined pill continuously by tricycling or extending the combined pill for longer than 21 days or shortening the hormone-free interval to four days is unlicensed but can be beneficial. The only licensed combined pill with a reduced hormone-free interval is Qlaira of two days and Zoely of four days. Extended use or tricycling is where three cycles of monophasic pills are taken in a row without a break. The hormone-free week is then taken at the end of the three months, and this is followed by a further three packets of pills. This reduces the number of pill-free weeks a woman has, so if she is complaining of problems in the hormone-free week, e.g. headaches, then this can reduce the number of headaches she experiences in a year.

When prescribing contraception out of its product license, it may be called unlicensed or off-label prescribing. This should be endorsed by expert opinion. The Faculty of Sexual and Reproductive Healthcare (2019, amended October 2023) supports tailored combined hormonal contraceptive regimes and recommends that women be aware of standard regimes and have information about tailored regimes. Women should be aware that tailored regimes are outside the product licence. The FSRH endorses the use of tailored regimes (FSRH, 2019, amended October 2023). Research shows that the use of tricycling, extended regimes and reduced hormone-free intervals have similar serious adverse incidents compared to regimens taken for 21 days with a 7-day hormone-free interval (FSRH, 2019, amended October 2023). In this situation, the prescriber takes the responsibility to monitor the patient and submit any suspected adverse reaction through the yellow card system (BNF, 2024). The woman should be involved in the decision and the course of treatment, alternative choices and why you are suggesting this regime. As a prescriber, you should not prescribe a drug that you have no experience with or is outside your area of competency. You should have evidence and knowledge of the drug and be able to justify your course of treatment (BNF, 2024).

The use of tailored regimes can be beneficial to women; however, this does not mean that these should be continuously prescribed without follow-up (Table 6.5).

Table 6.5 Table of tailored regimes (FSRH, 2019, amended October 2023)

Name of tailored and standard regimes	The length of the hormone-free interval	Description of tailored or standard regime. How long is the combined hormonal method used for?
Standard use	Seven-day hormone-free interval	21 days (21 active pills or 1 ring or 3 patches) are used.
Shortened hormone-free interval (HFI)	Four-day hormone-free interval	21 days (21 active pills or 1 ring or 3 patches).
Extended use (tricycling)	Four or seven days of hormone-free interval	9 weeks (3 × 21 active pills or 3 rings or 9 patches used consecutively).
Flexible extended use	Four days of hormone-free interval	Continuous use (≥21 days) of active pills, patches or rings until breakthrough bleeding (BTB) occurs for three to four days.
Continuous use	No hormone-free interval	Continuous use of active pills, patches or rings, none.

Side effects

- Nausea
- Headaches
- Breast tenderness and swelling
- BTB
- Mood swings
- Changes in libido
- Contact lenses may become uncomfortable – this is usually associated with hard lenses and high-dose pills

Decision of choice of pill

When commencing the client on the combined pill, the risks along with the benefits should be discussed fully so that the client is able to understand and weigh up the risks and benefits to them. Many women will initially be commenced on a second-generation combined pill, as these have less risk of a venous thromboembolism, but the risks between second- and third-generation pills needs to be discussed with the women. There are six low-dose combined pills all containing 20 mcg of oestrogen, all of which are third-generation pills: Mercilon, Gederal 20/150, Femodette, Millinette 20/75, Sunya 20/75 and Bimizza; however, there is no second-generation 20 mcg pill available. Some women will experience break through bleeding with 20 mcg combined pills and this is why most women will usually commence a 30 mcg second-generation combined pill.

Some women may be prescribed drospirenone containing pills such as Yasmin, Yacella, Yiznell, Lucette or Dretine; these are third-generation combined pills which contain 3 mg of drospirenone and 30 mcg of ethinylestradiol. Eloine is a third-generation combined pill which contains 3 mg of drospirenone and 20 mcg of ethinylestradiol. These are third-generation combined pills and have a higher risk of venous thrombosis, and this should be discussed along with second-generation combined pills with women.

Another type of combined pill is Qlaira, which contains oestradiol valerate and dienogest and has 26 active pills and 2 inactive pills; it has been found to reduce heavy menstrual bleeding and is the only combined pill licensed for this use. Qlaira's oestrogen is considered natural, and the progestogen dienogest is antiandrogenic. Qlaira has slightly different missed pill rules; a pill is missed if it is more than 12 hours late; then extra precautions will be required for 9 days.

Zoely is a combined pill which contains oestradiol and a progestogen, nomegestrol acetate; it has 28 pills, of which 24 are active pills and 4 are inactive. A pill is considered missed if it is more than 12 hours late, then extra precautions will be required for 7 days, and if these run into the inactive pills, these should be omitted and new active pills commenced. The Medicines and Healthcare Regulatory Authority (MHRA; FSRH, 2023e) have found that there is evidence of an increased risk of intracranial meningioma with nomegestrol acetate. However, this is with preparations which contain a higher dose of nomegestrol acetate and does not relate directly to Zoely. The FSRH (2023e) has advised that Zoely should not be taken by women with a current or past history of meningioma.

Many women are prescribed Dianette for acne treatment which contains 2 mg of cyproterone acetate and ethinylestradiol 35 mcg and provides contraception.

However, Dianette is not authorised for the sole purpose of contraception and should be discontinued after three or four menstrual cycles. There is evidence that Dianette has a higher incidence of venous thromboembolism (VTE) than in women using low-dose, oestrogen-containing combined pills (CSM, 2002) and is also associated with an increased risk of meningioma (FSRH, 2020). The MHRA and FSRH advise that individuals who have had a meningioma should not use any product containing cyproterone acetate. Women without a history of meningioma may use Co-cyprindiol/Dianette for management of acne/hirsutism, but clinicians should be vigilant for symptoms and signs of meningioma (FSRH, 2020). Many women are put on Dianette for the treatment of acne who would not normally be put on the combined pill because their BMI is over 30 or they have other contraindications. The reasons why a woman is taking Dianette should be reviewed and the risks discussed; many new low-dose combined pills give excellent contraception and improve acne with a lower risk of VTE.

DISCUSSING THE RISKS OF THE COMBINED PILL

The following risks should be discussed with all women considering the combined pill so that they are aware of the risks and anyone who is contraindicated is highlighted:

- VTE
- Arterial disease
- Breast cancer
- Migraines

Venous thromboembolism

There is a wide range of combined pills which may seem confusing when choosing a pill for a woman. The decision of which pill to prescribe will depend on the woman's medical and family history.

When explaining these risks to women, it is important to remember that women who are not on the combined pill have a risk of VTE of 2 in 10,000 per year, and even more importantly, the risk of VTE in pregnancy is 60 in 100, 000 per year (FSRH, 2019, amended 2023). The risks of VTE increase with age and obesity, along with other risk factors, are detailed next. So, whilst it is important to choose the right women to be on combined methods, it is also vital that the risks are explained clearly so that clients can understand these and the signs of VTE.

The range of combined pills used today is mainly divided into two groups known as second- and third-generation pills. Pills in Table 6.6 are second-generation pills and contain progestogens levonorgestrel, norethisterone or norgestimate, whilst the pills in Table 6.7 contain progestogens desogestrel, gestodene or drospirenone and are known as third-generation pills (FSRH, 2019, amended 2023).

The pill scare in 1995 was related to three epidemiological studies (Jick et al., 1995; WHO, 1995; Spitzer et al., 1996) which showed that pills containing progestogen levonorgestrel, norethisterone or ethynodiol (which is converted to norethisterone) have an incidence of VTE for women of 5–7 per 10, 000 per year (FSRH, 2019a, amended 2023). Women using combined contraceptive methods containing etonogestrel or norelgestromin found in the vaginal ring have a 5–7 in

Table 6.6 Second-generation pills: pills containing levonorgestrel, norethisterone or ethynodiol

Oestrogen content	20 mcg	30 mcg	35 mcg
		Loestrin 30	Ovysmen
		Microgynon	Norimin
		Ovranette	Brevinor
		Rigevidon	Norinyl-1
		Levest	
		Elevin	
		Ambelina	
		Levest	
		Maexeni	

Table 6.7 Third-generation pills: pills containing desogestrel, gestodene or drospirenone

Amount of ethinylestradiol	Gestodene	Desogestrel	Drospirenone
30 mcg	Femodene	Gederal 30/150	Dretine
	Femodene ED	Marvelon	Lucette
	Millinette 30/75	Cimizi	Yacella
	Katya 30/75		Yasmin
	Akizza		Yisnell
20 mcg	Akizza	Gederal 20/150	Eloine
	Femodette	Mercilon	
	Sunya	Bimizza	
	Millinette		

10,000 per year risk of venous thrombosis (FSRH, 2019, amended 2023). For women taking pills containing progestogens gestodene or desogestrel or drospirenone the incidence doubles to 9–12 in 10,000 per year (FSRH, 2019, amended 2023).

This research highlights the importance of selecting the right women for combined methods. No woman with a medical history of VTE should be prescribed the combined pill; this is an absolute contraindication. When assessing a woman's suitability for the pill, you should screen her for the following risk factors for VTE:

- Family history of VTE under the age of 45
- Prominent varicose veins
- Obesity (this is considered if the BMI is over 30 kg m^2)
- Immobility, e.g. wheelchair bound

When counselling a woman, you should discuss the research and risk factors related to the combined pill. Any woman with any risk factor for a VTE should, after discussion with her, either be changed to another method of contraception or changed to a pill with a lower risk of VTE, which would be a pill containing progestogens levonorgestrel, norethisterone or norgestimate (see Table 6.6); as always, a low-dose pill should be chosen.

Consultations should involve a comprehensive medical and family history; this is to identify women with inherited thrombophilia. Women on the combined oral contraceptive with mild thrombophilia, which includes factor V Leiden heterozygosity and prothrombin G20210A, mutations have a six times higher risk of a VTE than COC users without a thrombophilia mutation (FSRH, 2019, amended 2023). Whilst severe thrombophilia such as protein C and protein S deficiencies, antithrombin and the homozygous forms of V Leiden and prothrombin G20210A are associated with a seven-fold increased risk of VTE (FSRH, 2019, amended 2023). The FSRH has concluded that women with mild thrombophilia using combined contraception have an eight- to thirty-three-fold increase in VTE risk, and women with severe thrombophilia on combined methods have a seventy-fold increased risk of VTE (FSRH, 2019, amended 2023).

For men and women with a family history of inherited thrombophilia, screening is not accurate. A negative thrombophilia screen does not exclude a thrombophilia, and screening is generally of a low quality (FSRH, 2019, amended 2023). The FSRH recommends that women with a first-degree relative with an inherited thrombophilia be counselled and an alternative method to combined contraceptive methods be used (FSRH, 2019, amended 2023).

The Committee on Safety of Medicines advised that women who are intolerant to the second-generation pills but who are free of VTE risk factors may, if willing to accept the small increased risk of VTE, take the third-generation pill. Intolerance may be interpreted as minor side effects such as facial spots, acne or BTB which may be exacerbated by changing to a second-generation pill.

The risk of VTE is highest in the first few months of commencement of combined pills, and this reduces to the risk of non-users within weeks of discontinuation (FSRH, 2019, amended 2023). This highlights the risks women put themselves under by stopping and starting the combined pill for a few months, which some women do under the misconception that they are reducing the risks of it. Recent research by Meaidi et al. (FSRH, 2023d) suggests that for women taking hormonal contraception and using non-steroidal anti-inflammatory drugs (NSAID), the risk of venous thrombosis is higher although small. You should discuss this with your clients so that they are aware that NSAID drugs (often bought over the counter) could potentially increase VTE risk of combined contraception. As health professionals, it is important that we talk and answer questions about these risks and teach clients when to return early.

Arterial disease

Whilst it is important to assess women for risk factors for VTE it is equally important to assess for risk factors for arterial disease. Risk factors for arterial disease are as follows:

- Smoking
- Diabetes mellitus
- Mild to moderate hypertension, the combined pill is contraindicated if the diastolic blood pressure is above 95 mmHg
- Family history of arterial disease under the age of 45
- Obesity (BMI over 30 kg m^2)

You should discuss the risk factors for arterial disease with your client. If your client has more than one risk factor, then the combined pill will be contraindicated, and if she is over 35 and has any risk factors, then the COC should be discontinued. If there is any family history of arterial disease, you should encourage her to check her fasting lipids. Any family history of arterial disease under the age of 45 with no other risk factors necessitates relevant lipid screening. Research shows that the risk of arterial event is low with second- and third-generation combined pills, but there is limited data; however, the risk appears similar (FSRH, 2019, amended 2023). The risk of myocardial infarction and ischaemic stroke appears to be increased with combined pills containing higher 30–40 mcg doses of oestrogen; however, the risk remains small (FSRH, 2019, amended 2023).

When choosing a suitable combined pill, you should inform the woman of the risks so that she is able to make an informed decision. Medical histories should be updated regularly, and all issues discussed should be clearly documented and backed up with relevant information.

Migraines

It is important to ask all women about their headache and migraine history. Many women experience headaches which are in fact undiagnosed migraines, so it is important to highlight these women to identify which women are at an increased risk of an ischaemic stroke if they are given the combined pill. You will need to ask explicit questions, as the client may not be aware of the significance of her headaches; you may also find women who are taking the combined pills who are experiencing migraines with aura unaware of the risks. Questions like "Have you ever had a headache or migraine where you have experienced problems with your vision or had numbness or tingling?" usually help to reveal any past history. The United Medical Eligibility Criteria (FSRH, 2019a) states that if a woman suffers from one of the following types of migraine and she is already taking the combined pill or wishing to commence it, then she will have an absolute contraindication UKMEC 4 to it and will need to be reviewed by a doctor:

1 Migraine with aura; this is where there are focal neurological symptoms preceding the headaches. A woman might experience loss of vision or visual disturbances, numbness or tingling – this is UKMEC 4.
2 Migraine without aura where a woman has more than one additional risk factor for an ischaemic stroke. These additional risk factors include being 35 years of age and over, diabetes mellitus, family history of arterial disease below age of 45, hyperlipidaemia, hypertension, migraine, obesity (defined as a body mass index over 30), smoking and the combined pill. This is UKMEC 3/4.
3 Severe migraines which are severe and last longer than 72 hours.
4 Migraine which is treated with ergot derivatives.
5 Past history of migraine more than five years ago with aura is UKMEC 3.

Women with migraines have a two- to fourfold increased risk of an ischaemic stroke than women with migraines not taking combined contraception (FSRH, 2019a). It is important that women for whom you are not giving combined methods understand why you are refusing their request, so that they are not given it in the future if they go elsewhere.

Women who suffer from these types of migraines can use the progestogen-only pill, injectable or United Kingdom Medical Eligibility Criteria and any other non-hormonal method of contraception.

ACTIVITY

In the appendices of the UKMEC (FSRH, 2019), you will find links to the following resources. Have a look at these useful resources:

■ The Mayo Clinic has produced a video on migraine aura at http://www.mayoclinic.org/diseases-conditions/migraine-with-aura/multimedia/migraine-aura/vid-20084707
■ Information on headache classification can be found at The International Classification of Headache Disorders: https://ichd-3.org/

Breast cancer

The risk of breast cancer with the combined pill is small (FSRH, 2019, amended 2023). In June 1996, the Collaboration Group on Hormonal Factors in Breast Cancer published their study of re-analysis of world epidemiological data which related to 54 studies of over 53,000 women with breast cancer. Their re-analysis showed that there is a small increase in breast cancer risk for women taking the combined pill (Collaborative Group on Hormonal Factors in Breast Cancer, 1996a,b). The risk of breast cancer is when the woman is taking the combined pill, and in the ten years following cessation, there is a small increase in the relative risk of having breast cancer diagnosed. After ten years following stopping the combined pill, there is no increase in breast cancer risk. It was also found that women diagnosed with breast cancer who had used the COC had clinically less advanced cancers, which were less likely to have spread beyond the breast compared with those in women who had not used the combined pill. The risks of breast cancer were not associated with the dose, duration or any type of hormone in the combined pill. The results were the same for all ethnic groups, and for those with family histories of breast cancer and different reproductive histories (Faculty of Family Planning and Reproductive Health Care of the Royal College of Obstetricians and Gynaecologists, 1996). Because breast cancer incidence increases with age, the cumulative excess risk increases with increasing age for women starting and ten years after stopping the combined pill.

However, in 2002, studies by the US Centers for Disease Control and Prevention showed no increased combined pill–related risk of breast cancer (Marchbanks et al., 2002). Studies in 2010 also showed no increased risk of breast cancer (Vessey et al., 2010).

Recent research has shown that the increased risk of breast cancer is small but increased with duration (FSRH, 2019, amended 2023). However, data was unavailable for alcohol intake, age, menarche, feeding and incomplete for BMI. The Faculty of Sexual and Reproductive Healthcare advice is that any risk of breast cancer associated with the combined pill is small and will reduce after stopping it (2019, amended 2023). The risk of breast cancer with women taking the combined pill is small; this is a good opportunity to encourage women to self-examine their breasts and what to look for when doing so.

HOW TO TAKE THE COMBINED PILL

The combined 21-day pill should be commenced on the first day of your client's period. When she starts the pill on the first day of her period, no additional precautions are required; these instructions are the same for all 21-day pills, whether they are monophasic, or triphasic. If the pill is commenced at any other time in the cycle, additional precautions are required for seven days. You should encourage your client to take her pills at the same time each day. Once 21 days of pills have been taken, she should have a seven-day break where no pills are taken; this is known as the hormone-free week. Following the seven-day break she should restart the pill on day 8. Each packet of pills will always be commenced on the same day of the week the first packet is commenced.

Loss of efficacy of the combined pill

The combined pill's effectiveness is reduced by the following:

- Missed pills – if your client forgets to take her pill and is more than 48 hours late
- Vomiting – if your client vomits within three hours of taking the pill
- Severe diarrhoea
- Ulipristal acetate emergency contraception (UPA-EC) taken less than five days ago
- Drugs which are enzyme inducers (see Table 6.8)

Drug interactions

- Ulipristal Acetate Emergency contraception
  Combined hormonal contraception should not be quick started until five days after UPA-EC is taken as administration; this is because it is a progesterone receptor modulator and UPA-EC could reduce effectiveness of combined hormonal contraception (CHC).
- **Thyroxine**
  COC may increase requirement for thyroxine in some individuals with hypothyroidism by increasing thyroid binding globulin. There is limited research; however, it is advised that thyroid function is reviewed six weeks after commencing COC, as the thyroxine dose may need to be increased (FSRH, 2022).
- **Liver enzyme–inducing drugs**
  If your client is given an enzyme-inducing drug like rifampicin on a long-term basis, then alternative contraception is recommended, e.g. the injectable Depo-Provera given at ten-week intervals or an intrauterine device. Women wishing to continue with the combined pill whilst taking anticonvulsant or barbiturate

Table 6.8 Enzyme-inducing drugs which reduce the efficacy of combined methods by the induction of liver enzymes, which increase the metabolism of the combined methods. Up-to-date information on drug interactions can be found at **https://bnf.nice.org.uk/interactions/**

Drug type	*Drug*
Anticonvulsants	Carbamazepine Esilcarbamazepine Oxcarbazepine Fosphenytoin Phenytoin Perampanel Phenobarbital Primidone Topiramate Rufinamide
Antitubercle	Rifamycins, e.g. rifampicin, rifabutin
Antiretroviral – protease inhibitors	Ritonavir Ritonavir-boosted atazanavir Ritonavir-boosted tipranavir Ritonavir-boosted saquinavir Nelfinavir, darunavir, fosamprenavir, lopinavir
Antiretroviral – non-nucleoside reverse transcriptase inhibitors	Nevirapine Efavirenz
Other enzyme-inducing drugs	Modafinil Bosentan Aprepitant
Homeopathic	St John's Wort
Others	*Lamotrigine* (antiepileptic) and *griseofulvin* (antifungal). Contraceptive efficacy may be reduced by concurrent use of sugammadex

drugs, which affect the efficacy of the COC, will need to change to a pill containing a higher concentration of oestrogen – at least 50 g – and tricycle (this means taking three monophasic packets of pill in a row without a break). The hormone-free interval may also be decreased to four days to increase the efficacy of the pill. If BTB occurs, then the oestrogen content of the pill should be increased to 60–90 mcg once abnormal pathology has been excluded. It takes four weeks for the liver's excretory function to return to normal once liver enzyme drugs have been discontinued. It is advisable to allow eight weeks following cessation before a lower combined pill is commenced.

Lamotrigine is not thought to be an enzyme-inducing drug; however, the drug manufacturer advises that contraceptive effectiveness may be reduced. Serum levels of lamotrigine may be reduced when taking CHC, and this could result in reduced seizure control or lamotrigine toxicity (FSRH, 2022).

- **Liver enzyme–inhibiting drugs**

  Enzyme-inhibiting drugs which are taken with the CHC could result in elevated ethinylestradiol serum levels and potentially increased side effects such as venous thrombosis. Drugs that inhibit liver enzymes may increase the levels of hormones; these are detailed in Table 6.9.

Table 6.9 Enzyme-inhibiting drugs which increase hormonal contraception bioavailability and may increase risks of CHC. Up-to-date information on drug interactions can be found at **https://bnf.nice.org.uk/interactions/**

Antibacterials (e.g. erythromycin)
Antifungals (e.g. fluconazole, itraconazole, ketoconazole, posaconazole, voriconazole)
Antiretrovirals (e.g. atazanavir)
Immunosuppressants (e.g. tacrolimus)
Non-steroidal anti-inflammatories (e.g. etoricoxib)
Statins (e.g. atorvastatin, rosuvastatin)
Vasodilators (e.g. sitaxentan sodium)
Non-steroidal anti-inflammatories (e.g. etoricoxib)

MISSED PILL RULES

Many women either forget or are given little information about missed pill rules, so it is a good idea to check frequently that your client is up to date with current guidelines and has relevant written information to back this up. The importance of this information is often underestimated by both women and professionals; however, as poor compliance will affect the efficacy of the combined pill; it is essential that missed pill rules are covered.

If your client forgets a pill but it is within 24 hours from when she normally takes it, then she should take it immediately, and no additional precautions are required. However, if the pill is forgotten more than 24 hours but less than 72 hours from when it is normally taken, then the pill should be taken, and no additional precautions are required.

If your client forgets two or more pills, or it is now more than 72 hours late, then the missed pill should be taken, and the remaining pills taken at the normal time, but extra precautions will now be required for seven days. If the hormone-free interval runs into this time, then this should be omitted, and the next packet commenced straight away if it is a monophasic pill (see Figure 6.1). If the pill is triphasic and the pill-free week runs into this time, then the pill-free week should be omitted, but the client will need to take enough pills from the end of another packet which match the end of the present packet in colour and dose and take additional precautions for seven days following the missed pill. If the pill is an everyday (ED) pill and the seven days of additional precautions required run into the end of the packet, the seven inactive pills should be omitted and the next packet commenced straight away.

If the pills are missed in the first seven days of the packet and there has been unprotected sexual intercourse in the pill-free interval or in the first week of the packet, then emergency contraception should be considered. If the pills are missed in the second week of the packet days 8–14, then emergency contraception is not required if the pills have not been missed for the previous 7 days of the packet. Extra precautions will be required for the next seven days of pills.

If your client vomits within two hours of taking the pill or suffers from very severe diarrhoea, then the combined pill will not be effective, and additional precautions will be required during this time and for a further seven days once these symptoms have resolved. Again, if this runs into the hormone-free interval then this should be omitted, and if it is a monophasic pill, the next packet should be resumed immediately. If the pill is a triphasic pill, then your client will

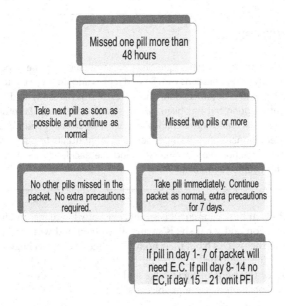

Figure 6.1 Missed combined oral contraceptive pill guidelines.

need to take enough pills from the end of another packet which match in dose and colour.

Women are safe to have sexual intercourse in the seven-day hormone-free interval if they do not lengthen this gap. If your client lengthens this gap, then she is at risk of ovulating and pregnancy. If she forgets the last pill of her packet, she should be advised to count that as the first day of the hormone-free interval and only have a further six pill-free days. If she forgets to restart her next packet on time and has had an eight-day pill-free interval, then her pills will not be contraceptively effective until she has taken seven days of pills; in the meantime, she will need to use additional contraceptive precautions. If she is more than one pill late in restarting her packet, then emergency contraception may be required.

INITIAL CONSULTATION

Time spent covering the risks and missed pill rules of the combined pill may alleviate future problems and save you and your client time and anxiety in the future. Many women attend having made their contraceptive choice; this does not mean that they do not have absolute contraindications to the combined pill, so a careful medical history of the client and her family is vital. Often, a change in contraception is precipitated by unprotected sexual intercourse or an accident with another contraceptive method, so it is important to establish whether emergency contraception is required. Details about the last menstrual period should be obtained, as this will help to build a picture of whether there is any possibility of pregnancy. If there has been unprotected sexual intercourse, then the client may already be pregnant, and a pregnancy test may need to be performed. Unprotected sexual intercourse is often abbreviated to UPSI.

CASE HISTORY 1

A 23-year-old woman consults requesting the combined pill. She appears aloof and distant, answering questions with limited replies and poor eye contact. When asked about previous contraception, she states she has recently had two years with no contraception but has been having sexual intercourse. Eventually, with time she says "that things have changed in her relationship," and although she wanted to get pregnant, she no longer does. The opportunity to discuss the problems within her relationship are discussed, and she decides to see if her partner will attend for couple counselling.

Look carefully at how your client is sitting, her body language, and listen to how she is talking to you and what she is saying. Both men and women can tell you a great deal about themselves from their body language and the feelings they portray.

The risks of the combined pill should be discussed. It is important that your client is aware of the signs of these risks and when to attend early. If your client experiences any of the following problems she should seek medical attention:

- Pain and swelling in the calf of her leg
- Chest pain
- Shortness of breath
- Increasing headaches
- Headaches with speech or visual disturbances
- Pain, tingling or weakness in an arm or leg
- Jaundice
- Severe abdominal pain
- Post-coital bleeding or any prolonged bleeding

Basic observations should be performed like blood pressure, weight, and height. You should calculate your client's BMI, which will help to exclude any absolute contraindications. Details of previous contraception should be covered with any problems your client encountered, as this will help you choose a suitable pill for your client.

Missed pill rules and emergency contraception should be covered, along with when to commence the pill and when efficacy is reduced. Often, women do not know how long after unprotected sexual intercourse emergency contraception may be given, and even if they never need to use this information, they may have a friend who does. What is often forgotten is that women learn a great deal from their friends, but sometimes this information is inaccurate; on many occasions, a client's visit is prompted by a friend.

During your history taking, you will eliminate any absolute contraindications to the pill. If there are signs of vaginal infection, then appropriate screening should be performed; if this is unavailable, then she should be referred to a genitourinary medicine clinic. If your client is experiencing any post-coital bleeding (often abbreviated to PCB), then she should be referred for a cervical smear along with a bimanual examination. PCB can be a sign of infection, cervical ectopy, polyps, or malignancy. If there are no problems, then you should record previous cervical cytology and discuss with your client when this needs to be repeated. Women who have not had a cervical smear often fear being forced to have a smear, but if there are no clinical problems, then this may be deferred to a convenient time. If your client has any sexual anxieties or problems, then she may feel comfortable discussing them nearer the end of the consultation. Giving time and allowing her to talk will help enable her to approach this difficult subject.

This is a prime time to discuss disease prevention. If your client has a family history of heart disease, then it can be useful to discuss blood lipid screening, diet, and smoking. You should discuss with your client how the risks of the pill are increased by smoking; if she ceases smoking, then these risks will reduce to the same of a non-smoker. It is also a good opportunity to promote breast awareness, and preconceptual screening such as sickle cell screening and rubella status. Although your client may have no intention now of becoming pregnant, this is often a good time to perform screening in case immunisation for rubella is required.

Women often underestimate the need for protection against sexually transmitted infections and HIV. There is a belief among many men and women that "it won't happen to me," and it is often difficult for a nurse to approach this subject when clients are unable to accept this is an issue. However, you will need to discuss safer sex and the use of condoms with your client, as the pill offers no protection against STIs and HIV, and she may not have considered this subject.

Discuss with your client initial problems she may encounter and how to alleviate these, e.g. BTB and nausea (see the section "Problems Encountered on the Pill") and when you will need to see her again. It is important to inform your client of any potential side effects, as this will help alleviate anxiety. Most side effects normally settle within the first three months, so it is always worth continuing with a pill rather than changing to another pill where the symptoms may be perpetuated. A woman commencing the combined pill should be seen in three months' time. If there are no problems, then she should be seen every six months from then onwards.

Lastly, everything you have discussed with your client should be backed up with up-to-date written information. Often, men and women do not read leaflets, so you cannot rely on just giving the leaflets – you need to say it verbally as well. It is also possible that your client is unable to read but may not be prepared to admit this, or English is not her first language. If this is the case, try to obtain leaflets in her first language. You should also give telephone numbers where clients can obtain advice and emergency contraception.

CASE HISTORY 2

A 26-year-old woman consults, having been on the combined pill for five years. She complains of increased headaches, and on discussion, she says that she is experiencing visual problems with the headaches. When she reads with her headache, she finds that she is unable to see words in the text and has been getting some tingling in her tongue. It is explained to the client that what she is experiencing are focal migraines, and these are an absolute contraindication with the combined pill and put her at an increased risk of a stroke. After discussion with the client, other methods of contraception are discussed, and the client decides to try the progestogen pill and is given Cerazette whilst she considers other methods. She is now unable to take the combined pill, patch or ring as her headaches are focal migraines and this is an absolute contraindication to these methods as they contain oestrogen, but she may be given progestogen methods.

Subsequent visits

At subsequent visits, it is important to ascertain whether your client has had any problems of any kind, which may include increasing headaches or migraines. This may be performed by asking open-ended questions like, "How have you got on with your pill?" Allow her time to answer questions. Often, clients report that they have no problems, but just as they are about to leave mention that they have had visual problems with a headache or forgotten a pill or not used extra precautions.

Routine observations of weight, BMI and blood pressure should be performed. Information about the last menstrual period will help eliminate any risk of pregnancy and checks that she is taking her pills correctly. Is your client's cervical smear up to date; is she experiencing any problems with her periods or sexual intercourse? Is your client aware of missed pill rules and emergency contraception, does she have up-to-date information? Does she have any anxieties or questions?

Does she need a supply of condoms, is she aware of how to apply a condom or does she need to be taught? A prescription of 12 months or supply if your trust allows this in Patient Group Directives (PGDs) may be given. If your client is a non-smoker and has no contraindications or complications, then she may continue to take the pill until she is perimenopausal.

ACTIVITY

Do you know where your clients can obtain contraception and emergency contraception in your area when you are not working?

Reasons for breakthrough bleeding with the COC

It is not unusual for women to have BTB in the first two months of starting a combined pill; this can be alarming for women if they are not warned beforehand of this possibility. It is important that women continue to take their pill as the bleeding usually stops after two to three packets and, providing all the pills have been taken correctly, contraceptive efficacy will not be affected. If bleeding continues beyond three packets of pills, then the cause should be investigated, which may be due to the following:

- Missed pills
- Diarrhoea or vomiting
- Drugs which interact with the COC and affect the efficacy, e.g. enzyme-inducing drugs
- Disease of the cervix, e.g. cervical cancer, sexually transmitted infections such as chlamydia
- Pregnancy
- Diet, e.g. vegetarians
- The dose of the pill may not suit the client

When excluding all possible causes of BTB, it is vital to take a detailed history from the woman. This will help ascertain what the cause is and whether contraceptive efficacy has been reduced, and emergency contraception is indicated. The type of pill preparation should not be changed until all causes have been excluded. If the BTB is caused by the dose of pill preparation, then a pill with a different or higher dose of progestogen should be prescribed.

PROBLEMS ENCOUNTERED ON THE PILL

■ BREAKTHROUGH BLEEDING:

BTB may be due to disease of the cervix, such as cervical neoplasia, or a sexually transmitted infection, such as chlamydia, so appropriate screening may need to be performed. Pregnancy may cause BTB, so this may need to be excluded. If your client has missed pills, had diarrhoea or vomiting, then there may be loss of effectiveness of the pill and bleeding. Drugs which cause loss of efficacy of the pill may cause BTB (see Table 6.8). The client may need to change to alternative contraception or change to a higher oestrogen content pill. Women who are vegetarians occasionally have BTB, as their enterohepatic circulation may be affected by their bowel flora. Occasionally, women who have had extensive bowel surgery may suffer BTB because the absorption of the pill is impaired.

BTB may occur because your client has not been on the pill for a long enough duration. It is not unusual to experience BTB in the first few months of taking the pill; this usually disappears, so it is important to continue with the pill. However, if bleeding is experienced and she has taken the pill for three to four packets with no improvement, and all other causes of BTB have been excluded, then the dosage or type of pill may need to be changed. The pill may be changed, as the dose of it may be too low; this can be done by choosing a pill with a higher oestrogen content or one with a different progestogen component. It may be necessary to prescribe a pill containing 50 mcg of oestrogen.

■ YOUR CLIENT FORGETS TO TAKE HER PILL:

It is useful to discuss with your client why she thinks she forgets her pills; this may be because of problems in a relationship, or she may subconsciously desire a pregnancy. If she forgets her pill, it can be a useful reminder to keep the pill by her alarm clock, or by the coffee or tea jar, or by her toothbrush or she could set her phone to remind her. It is a good idea to suggest she carries a spare packet of the pill in her purse so if she has forgotten to take her pill, she is likely to have the packet with her. Alarm watches, personal computers and mobile phones can be set to act as a reminder. There are apps that can be downloaded to help remind clients about pill taking.

■ COMPLAINTS OF NAUSEA:

If your client complains of nausea, she should make sure that the pill is taken after eating. If this continues, she may need to change to a different type of pill or one containing less oestrogen.

■ BREAST TENDERNESS:

If this is experienced in the first three months, then usually the symptoms resolve. However, if your client complains of breast tenderness, her breasts should be examined. Evening primrose oil and vitamin B6 can help relieve symptoms if taken continuously. If symptoms persist, it may be necessary to change to a pill containing lower levels of oestrogen and progestogen or a different type of progestogen.

- INCREASED SPOTS AND ACNE:
    Try changing to a pill with a different progestogen.
- WEIGHT GAIN:
    Often, clients complain of increased weight. Initially they may have a small weight gain, but usually weight gain is due to changes in diet and exercise.
- VAGINAL DRYNESS AND LOSS OF LIBIDO:
    Try to discuss with her any anxieties or problems she may have in the relationship which may be causing this problem. Try changing to a different pill.
- HEADACHES PRIOR TO PERIODS:
    It is important to check that these headaches do not cause focal disturbances, as this would be an absolute contraindication to the pill. It may be useful for your client to keep a diary of her headaches and when they occur. If they occur in the hormone-free interval, then tricycling will reduce the number of headaches. Headaches in the pill-free week are usually because the hormone levels have dropped.

Combined transdermal patch

Introduction and history

The first combined transdermal patch was launched on to the UK market in 2003. There is only one combined transdermal patch currently available, known as Evra from Janssen-Cilag. The transdermal patch is only provided in one skin colour pale pink, currently there is a campaign "Clap Back on the Contraceptive Patch," which is aimed at manufactures to provide the transdermal patch in different skins tones making the patch more fairer to all women (FSRH, 2023f).

Explanation of the method

Evra releases 150 micrograms of norelgestromin and 20 micrograms of ethinylestradiol per 24 hours; norelgestromin is the primary active metabolite of norgestimate. Evra is a transdermal patch which lasts seven days. A patch is used for three weeks, changed each week with a new patch and followed by a hormone-free interval of seven days in the fourth week where a withdrawal bleed occurs. Evra prevents pregnancy by inhibiting ovulation, altering cervical mucus so that it is impenetrable to sperm and making the endometrium unfavourable to implantation.

Efficacy

The efficacy for combined transdermal patch is over 99% with careful and consistent use; however, with less careful use it can be 91% (FSRH, 2019, amended 2023). There is limited evidence to suggest that in women whose weight is equal to or greater than 90 kg, contraceptive efficacy may be decreased (FSRH, 2019, amended 2023).

UKMEC 4 unacceptable health risk – absolute contraindication

Contraindications are the same for combined transdermal patch as with the combined pill.

- Pregnancy
- Breast feeding
- Less than six weeks post-partum
- Undiagnosed vaginal or uterine bleeding
- Past or present venous thrombosis
- Past or present arterial thrombosis
- Cardiovascular and ischaemic heart disease
- Complicated pulmonary hypertension, atrial fibrillation, and subacute bacterial endocarditis
- Cardiomyopathy with impaired cardiac function
- Migraine with aura
- Cerebrovascular accident and transient ischaemic attacks
- Active disease of the liver, e.g. malignancy, hepatocellular adenoma, history of cholestatic jaundice, impaired liver function tests, acute viral hepatitis, severe compensated cirrhosis
- Current breast cancer
- Positive antiphospholipid antibodies
- Raynaud's disease with lupus anticoagulant, if present, will increase coagulation
- Stevens–Johnson syndrome
- Acute pancreatitis
- Known thrombogenic mutations such as factor V Leiden, prothrombin mutation, protein S and protein C and Antithrombin deficiencies
- Smokers over the age of 35
- Hypertension with a systolic of 160 mmHg or diastolic over 100 mmHg
- Prolonged immobility

UKMEC 3 risks outweigh the benefits of using method – relative contraindication.

- Obesity (BMI over 35 kg m^2)
- Lipid disorders and diseases where HDL is reduced, e.g. diabetes, hypertension
- Migraine without aura
- History of migraine with aura, which was more than five years ago, at any age
- History of migraine with aura more than five years ago
- Multiple risk factors for cardiovascular disease
- Hypertension with a systolic over 140–159 mmHg or diastolic over 90–99 mmHg
- Severe diabetes mellitus with complications such as retinopathy, neuropathy, vascular disease
- Carriers of known gene mutations linked to breast cancer BRCAS 1/BRCAS 2
- Past history of breast cancer initiation needs to be in discussion with oncology team
- History of cholestasis with a combined method
- Current and medically treated gallbladder disease

- Diseases whose drug treatment affects the efficacy of the combined pill, e.g. tuberculosis, epilepsy
- Complicated organ transplant
- Family history of arterial or venous disease in a first-degree relative below the age of 45
- Immobility

Side effects

- Nausea
- Breast tenderness and swelling
- Headache
- Application site skin reactions

How to take the combined transdermal patch

The combined transdermal patch should be commenced initially on the first day of a woman's menstrual period. The patch should be applied to clean dry hairless skin; the patch should be held down firmly for about 10 seconds until firmly attached. The site of the patch should be changed each week. The patch should remain *in situ* for seven days; a new patch should be applied on day 8 and this should remain *in situ* for a further seven days. A new patch should be applied on day 15; this is the third patch that remains applied until day 22 when the patch is removed and there is a hormone-free interval for seven days. During these seven days, a withdrawal bleed occurs; a new patch is applied on day 8.

Loss of efficacy of the combined transdermal patch

The combined transdermal patch's effectiveness is reduced by the following:

- Patch comes off or is partly detached, or late changing or commencing of a new patch
- Combined hormonal contraception should not be quick started until five days after UPA-EC is taken as this is because it is a progesterone receptor modulator and UPA could reduce effectiveness of CHC
- Drugs which are enzyme inducers (see Table 6.8)

Loss of efficacy through drug interaction

The effectiveness of the combined transdermal patch is reduced with enzyme-inducing drugs; see Table 6.8.

Missed patch rules

If a patch detaches for less than 48 hours, then it should be re-applied or replaced with a new patch immediately and no additional contraception is applied.

The next patch should be changed on the usual change day. If the patch has been detached for 48 hours or more, then a new contraceptive patch should be applied and new cycle commenced; additional contraception is required for seven days. If the patch was in week 1, then emergency contraception will be required for any unprotected sexual intercourse.

If the patch change day is delayed in week 2 or 3 by 48 hours or more, the client should apply a new patch immediately. The next patch should be applied on the usual patch change day; if the patch has been worn correctly for the seven preceding days, emergency contraception is not required. If the patch change is prior to the hormone-free interval, then this should be omitted and condoms used for seven days.

COMBINED VAGINAL RING.

Introduction and history

The combined vaginal ring was launched in the UK in January 2009 and is manufactured by Organon under the name NuvaRing.

Explanation of the method

The combined vaginal ring is a non-biodegradable latex-free combined contraceptive vaginal ring which releases in 24 hours 120 micrograms of the progestogen etonogestrel and 15 micrograms of the oestrogen ethinylestradiol and remains in the vagina for three weeks. It is then removed for one week when a withdrawal bleed will occur, and then a new ring is inserted. The combined vaginal ring is 4 mm thick and 54 mm in diameter and can be inserted into the vagina and removed by women.

The combined vaginal ring prevents pregnancy by inhibiting ovulation, altering cervical mucus so that it is impenetrable to sperm and by making the endometrium unfavourable to implantation.

Efficacy

The efficacy for the combined vaginal ring is over 99% with careful and consistent use; however, with less careful use it can be 91% (FSRH, 2019, amended 2023).

UKMEC 4 unacceptable health risk – absolute contraindication

Contraindications are the same for the combined vaginal ring as with the combined pill.

- Pregnancy
- Breast feeding
- Less than six weeks post-partum

- Undiagnosed vaginal or uterine bleeding
- Past or present venous thrombosis
- Past or present arterial thrombosis
- Cardiovascular and ischaemic heart disease
- Complicated pulmonary hypertension, atrial fibrillation, and subacute bacterial endocarditis
- Cardiomyopathy with impaired cardiac function
- Migraine with aura
- Cerebrovascular accident and transient ischaemic attacks
- Active disease of the liver, e.g. malignancy, hepatocellular adenoma, history of cholestatic jaundice, impaired liver function tests, acute viral hepatitis, severe compensated cirrhosis
- Current breast cancer
- Positive antiphospholipid antibodies
- Raynaud's disease with lupus anticoagulant if present this will increase coagulation
- Stevens–Johnson syndrome
- Acute pancreatitis
- Known thrombogenic mutations such as factor V Leiden, prothrombin mutation, protein S and protein C and Antithrombin deficiencies
- Smokers over the age of 35
- Hypertension with a systolic of 160 mmHg or diastolic over 100 mmHg
- Prolonged immobility

UKMEC 3 risks outweigh the benefits of using method – relative contraindication

- Obesity (BMI over 35 kg m^2)
- Lipid disorders and diseases where HDL is reduced, e.g. diabetes, hypertension
- Migraine without aura
- History of migraine with aura, which was more than five years ago, at any age
- History of migraine with aura more than five years ago
- Multiple risk factors for cardiovascular disease
- Hypertension with a systolic over 140–159 mmHg or diastolic over 90–99 mmHg
- Severe diabetes mellitus with complications such as retinopathy, neuropathy, vascular disease
- Carriers of known gene mutations linked to breast cancer BRCAS 1/BRCAS 2
- Past history of breast cancer initiation needs to be in discussion with oncology team
- History of cholestasis with a combined method
- Current and medically treated gallbladder disease
- Diseases whose drug treatment affects the efficacy of the combined pill, e.g. tuberculosis, epilepsy
- Complicated organ transplant

- Family history of arterial or venous disease in a first-degree relative below the age of 45
- Immobility

How to use the combined vaginal ring

Combined vaginal ring should be inserted into the vagina on the first day of the period and left *in situ* for three weeks; this should be followed by a seven-day hormone-free interval, after which a new ring should be inserted for a further three weeks. Combined vaginal ring will be effective in preventing pregnancy if started on the first day of the period; if started from day 2 of the cycle onwards extra precautions will be required for seven days. During the ring-free week, women should experience a withdrawal bleed. Women should be shown how to remove and fit the ring; the ring should be compressed and inserted into the vagina; it does not need to be in a particular position but should feel comfortable. To remove the ring, women should loop their finger around the ring and pull it out. The ring should be disposed of in household waste.

The ring's position should be checked prior to intercourse to check that it is correctly positioned. The combined vaginal ring may be left *in situ* during sexual intercourse and if tampons are used.

Prior to dispensing the combined vaginal ring, it should be kept in a pharmacy fridge at temperatures between 2°C and 8°C and can be stored this way for 40 months. Once the combined vaginal ring is dispensed, it can be left out of the fridge for four months, because of this, only three months of the combined vaginal ring can be dispensed at a time. When the three-month pack is dispensed, the date should be written and the lifespan outside the fridge should be discussed. Women should keep their combined vaginal rings at room temperature once dispensed. A prescription can be given for a further three months so that women can obtain this from the chemist when they need it.

Loss of efficacy of the combined vaginal ring

As the etonogestrel and ethinylestradiol in the ring are absorbed via the vagina, they avoid the first pass metabolism of oral combined methods and so will not be affected by gastrointestinal disturbances and malabsorption disorders from the upper bowel. However, the antifungal drug miconazole has been shown to increase the release of etonogestrel and ethinylestradiol resulting in higher serum levels. Antifungals do not appear to reduce contraceptive efficacy; however, they are associated with increase in ring breakages (FSRH, 2009b).

Loss of efficacy through drug interaction

The effectiveness of the combined vaginal ring is reduced with enzyme-inducing drugs (see Table 6.8).

The combined vaginal ring should not be quick started until 5 days after UPA-EC is taken; this is because it is a progesterone receptor modulator and UPA could reduce effectiveness of CHC.

Missed combined vaginal ring rules

The combined vaginal ring's efficacy can be reduced if the ring is left out of the vagina for more than 48 hours; extra precautions should be advised for seven days. If this is in the first week of the ring, then emergency contraception will be required for any unprotected sexual intercourse. If the ring has been left out of the vagina, and it is in the second and third weeks of use, and the ring has been used consistently in the last seven days, then only extra precautions will be required for seven days. If in week 3, the woman can insert a new ring and miss her hormone-free interval.

If the hormone-free interval is lengthened beyond 21 days to 28 days, no extra precautions are required. Start a hormone-free interval if scheduled and insert a new ring at the end of the HFI.

Sexuality and anxieties

The combined contraception has given women a greater freedom over their bodies and fertility. The pill has allowed women to choose when they wish to become pregnant. However, this has drawbacks: women often find the decision to stop the pill and try to conceive a dilemma. They hope to find the perfect time to become pregnant, which will probably never happen; at the same time, they feel that time is running out as their body clock ticks ominously away! For some women, the pill is too effective; they would like to become pregnant and not have to make the decision.

Women who frequently forget to take their pill may have a subconscious desire to become pregnant, but it may be difficult for them to admit this feeling. Some women have been brought up to believe that sexual intercourse is only for procreation, and by taking the pill, they are preventing pregnancy, resulting in loss of enjoyment of sexual intercourse.

Women may blame the combined pill for problems which are unrelated to it. Frequent changes of type of pill may indicate an underlying problem. Given time and an empathetic approach, these may be vocalised.

Some women feel an enormous amount of guilt for enjoying sexual intercourse with the protection of the pill, and this guilt is often expressed by women who feel that the pill will make them infertile. They feel that there is some divine retribution for being on the pill, and this has been compounded by pill scares. Recently, women and their partners have had to read and listen to alarmist articles and news reports in the UK about the pill; the anxiety this has engendered has been enormous. Articles entitled "The Pill Can Kill" have meant that many women now have a negative image of the combined pill which does not reflect the true properties of it. Women are often surprised at how small the risk of venous thromboembolism and breast cancer is! There is also the belief that there should be no risk attached to the pill. This unrealistic view fails to acknowledge the risks of pregnancy and the everyday risks we all automatically accept like driving a car or smoking. It is therefore important that we educate and inform women about the risks of the combined pill and can confront the anxieties and alarm they have in a calm and responsible manner.

SELF-ASSESSMENT QUESTIONS

Answers and discussion at the end of the chapter.

1 In what situations would extra precautions be required with the combined pill?
2 Name four beneficial effects the combined pill has on a woman's body.
3 What are the main concerns or myths about the combined pill that women worry about, and how would you answer their questions?
4 Name the second-generation pills missing in the table below; see Table 6.6 for answers on page xx.
5 Name the third-generation pills missing in the table below; see Table 6.7 for answers on page xx (Tables 6.10 and 6.11).

Table 6.10 Name the second-generation combined pill under their correct oestrogen content

Oestrogen content	20 mcg	30 mcg	35 mcg	Phasic

Table 6.11 Name the third-generation combined pill

	Gestodene	Desogestrel	Drospirenone
30			3 mg
20			

ANSWERS TO SELF-ASSESSMENT QUESTIONS

1 In what situations would extra precautions be required with the combined pill?
    Extra precautions are required when the pill's effectiveness is decreased. This may be due to a pill being taken more than 48 hours late from its normal time. Extra precautions are also required if the woman has severe diarrhoea or vomiting or commences a drug which reduces the efficacy of the pill like an enzyme-inducing drug, e.g. rifampicin.

2　Name four beneficial effects the combined pill has on a woman's body.

The combined pill reduces the risk of endometrial and ovarian cancer. It reduces benign breast disease, dysmenorrhoea and menorrhagia, and because of this, it reduces the incidence of iron deficiency anaemia. There is less risk of ectopic pregnancies and a reduction of functional ovarian cysts. Psychologically, the combined pill gives women assurance against unwanted pregnancy and relief of possible disabling pre-menstrual symptoms.

3　What are the main concerns or myths about the combined pill that women worry about, and how would you answer their questions?

One of the major concerns that women wish to discuss about the combined pill which is a myth is that "the pill makes you infertile." The pill is completely reversible and does not cause infertility (FSRH, 2019, amended 2023); however, no one knows whether they can become pregnant until they do so. A study on primary infertility and the combined pill (Bagwell et al., 1995) concluded that the COC was associated with a lower incidence of primary infertility.

Another concern women have is related to the length of time they take the pill; they feel "you should give your body a rest from the pill." There is no medical reason to stop the pill. Often, when women do stop to have a rest, this is when they accidentally become pregnant, causing them great anguish.

Many women are concerned that the pill is dangerous. In fact, the combined pill is a very safe and effective form of contraception. It is not dangerous unless there is a medical contraindication. Smoking is more of a health risk than taking the pill, which is why smokers cannot have the pill after the age of 35.

PROGESTOGEN METHODS

7

INTRODUCTION

Progestogen only methods comprise of progestogen-only-pills, progestogen-only-injectables and progestogen only implants.

PROGESTOGEN PILLS

Introduction and history

The progestogen-only pill (POP) used to be referred to as the "mini pill," which tends to give women the impression that it is of a low contraceptive efficacy. There are three groups of POPs: traditional POPs which contain the progestogens levonorgestrel (LNG) or norethisterone (NET), desogestrel POPs and drospirenone progestogen-only pills. Table 7.2 outlines traditional POPs, and Table 7.1 outlines desogestrel POPs and drospirenone POPs. Progestogen pills have many advantages over other methods which are often not recognised.

EXPLANATION OF THE METHOD

- The desogestrel progestogen pills primary method of preventing pregnancy is inhibition of ovulation (FSRH, August 2022a, amended July 2023). Desogestrel and drospirenone pills also thicken the cervical mucus, and thin the endometrium and reduce fallopian tube motility.
- The traditional progestogen pill (POP) prevents pregnancy in a number of ways by thickening the cervical mucus hindering sperm penetrability; they also render the endometrium unreceptive for implantation and reduce fallopian tube function. In some cycles, ovulation is suppressed.

EFFICACY

If used carefully and consistently, all progestogen pills are more than 99% effective in preventing pregnancy. For typical use, the efficacy will be lower; this may be due to women not taking their pills on time (referred to as user error).

The research surrounding the efficacy of progestogen pills and which group is more effective is limited, so it is difficult to ascertain whether there is a significant difference (FSRH, August 2022a, amended July 2023).

DOI: 10.4324/9781003484424-8

Evidence suggests that progestogen pills are not affected by weight or BMI, and there is no evidence to suggest supporting doubling the dose of progestogen pill (FSRH, August 2022a, amended July 2023).

PHARMACOKINETICS AND PHARMACODYNAMICS

Progestogens are absorbed in the small intestine and metabolised in the liver and excreted in faeces. There is no enterohepatic recirculation of progestogens, so efficacy is unchanged by changes to gut flora (FSRH, 2022b). Absorption of progestogens will be affected by severe diarrhoea and vomiting. Drugs that may affect absorption include chelating drugs and drugs that alter gastric pH. Metabolism of progestogens will be affected by cytochrome P450 enzymes that are induced by certain drugs, as seen in Table 7.3.

ADVANTAGES

- Does not inhibit lactation, so suitable for breast feeding
- No evidence of increased risk of cardiovascular disease
- No evidence of increased risk of venous thromboembolism
- No evidence of increased risk of hypertension
- Does not need to be stopped prior to surgery
- Suitable for women with diabetes or focal migraines
- Reduction in dysmenorrhoea
- May relieve premenstrual symptoms
- Suitable for women unable to take oestrogen

DISADVANTAGES

- Needs to be taken carefully to be effective
- Irregular menstrual cycle
- A small number of women develop functional ovarian cysts
- If POP fails, may have possible increased ectopic pregnancy rate

UKMEC 4 unacceptable health risk – absolute contraindications

- Current breast cancer
- Pregnancy
- Allergy to a constituent. The manufacturer advises that the drospirenone (DRSP) POP should not be used by individuals with severe renal insufficiency or acute renal failure. FSRH advise that individuals with known hyperkalaemia or untreated hypoaldosteronism (e.g. Addison's disease) or currently using potassium-sparing diuretics, aldosterone antagonists or potassium supplements should avoid DRSP pills (FSRH, August 2022a, amended July 2023)

UKMEC 3 risks outweigh the benefits of using method – relative contraindication

- History of breast cancer (the decision to commence any progestogen pills should be made in consultation with oncology team; FSRH, 2016 amended 2019)
- Current history of ischaemic heart disease, including cerebrovascular accident

and transient ischaemic attack whilst taking progestogen methods, needs to be reviewed
- Present liver disease, liver adenoma or cancer, severe decompensated liver cirrhosis
- Drugs which interfere with the efficacy of the POP, e.g. enzyme-inducing drugs
- Acute porphyrias
- Breast cancer, arterial thromboembolism that occurred during use of a POP, decompensated cirrhosis and hepatocellular tumours are UKMEC3 or UKMEC4 conditions for use of all POPs

RANGE OF METHOD

The progestogen-only pill contains the same amount of progestogen throughout the packet and is taken every day. Desogestrel progestogen pills are made of the progestogen desogestrel, and there are eight in the range; see Table 7.1.

There are two traditional progestogen pills: one is made of the progestogen norethisterone, and one is made of the progestogen levonorgestrel (Table 7.2). There is one drospirenone progestogen pill called Slynd® (Table 7.1).

Table 7.1 Desogestrel and drospirenone POPs

Pill type	Preparation	Manufacturer	Micrograms per pill	Type of progestogen
Cerazette	28-day pill	Organon	75 mcg	**Desogestrel**
Cerelle	28-day pill	Consilent Health Ltd	75 mcg	**Desogestrel**
Desomono	28-day pill	MedRx Licences Ltd	75 mcg	**Desogestrel**
Desorex	28-day pill	Somex Pharma	75 mcg	**Desogestrel**
Feanolla	28-day pill	Lupin Healthcare	75 mcg	**Desogestrel**
Moonia	28-day pill	Stragen Ltd	75 mcg	**Desogestrel**
Zelleta	28-day pill	Morningside Healthcare	75 mcg	**Desogestrel**
Desogestrel non-proprietary	28-day pill		75 mcg	**Desogestrel**
Drospirenone				
Slynd®	24 consecutive daily 4 mg drospirenone pills followed by four inactive pills	Exeltis healthcare S.L.	4 mg	**Drospirenone**

Table 7.2 Traditional POPs

Pill type	Preparation	Manufacturer	Micrograms per pill	Type of progestogen
Noriday	28-day pill	Pfizer	350 mcg	**Norethisterone**
Norgeston	35-day pill	Bayer	30 mcg	**Levonorgestrel**

DECISION OF CHOICE

As no research has found any difference in efficacy between the progestogen pills preparations, then the most suitable choice between them is the one which gives your client fewer side effects and less irregular bleeding. Desogestrel (DSG) progestogen pills have a larger window for missed pills, and the primary mode of action is to inhibit ovulation in comparison to LNG and NET progestogen pills and so should be the first line of treatment. Research on desogestrel pills comparing LNG pills (Rice et al., 1999; Collaborative Study Group, 1998) has shown desogestrel (DSG) pills in the form of Cerazette to have a significant inhibition of ovulation. Cerazette users had a higher incidence of amenorrhoea and infrequent bleeding, although some users had frequent bleeding and prolonged bleeding at the beginning of the study.

Drospirenone (DRSP) is a spironolactone derivative, as an aldosterone antagonist, it opposes aldosterone activity in the distal nephron, increasing potassium reuptake and increasing sodium and water excretion. As a result, hyperkalaemia has been observed in a few women taking DRSP POP (FSRH, August 2022a, amended July 2023). It is recommended that individuals with significant risk factors for chronic kidney disease have bloods for urea and electrolytes and blood pressure checked prior to prescription of the DRSP POP, particularly if aged over 50 years (FSRH, August 2022a, amended July 2023).

Progestogen pills efficacy is not affected by weight or BMI; there is no evidence to support increasing the dose (FSRH, August 2022a, amended July 2023). Women who undergo bariatric surgery should be advised that there is insufficient evidence about the efficacy of progestogen oral pills and should be advised to use a method which is not taken orally.

There have been concerns about the progestogen injectable Depo-Provera and osteoporosis; however, there are no concerns about other progestogen methods; however, data is limited (FSRH, August 2022a, amended July 2023). If a woman is a long-term user of the POP, has amenorrhoea and complains of hot flashes and vaginal dryness, then she should be investigated to see if she is menopausal.

Breast cancer is a hormone-dependent cancer, so taking any hormones may worsen current or recent breast cancer in a woman. There is no definitive research on the combined pill or progestogen methods; however, going on the worst-case scenario, the 1996 Collaborative Group on hormonal factors in breast cancer (Collaborative Group, 1996a, 1996b) found that the risk of breast cancer was similar to that of the combined pill, whilst other studies have showed no increased risk. The available evidence does not support an association between breast cancer and progestogen pills; however, any risk cannot be excluded due to limited research (FSRH, August 2022a, amended July 2023). Any risk is likely to be small; this is an area where the risk is unclear. All women should be encouraged to practice breast self-awareness and seek advice early from their general practitioner if they find any changes in their breasts.

SIDE EFFECTS

- Functional ovarian cysts
- Breast tenderness
- Bloatedness
- Depression
- Fluctuations in weight

- Nausea
- Irregular bleeding
- Amenorrhoea

HOW TO TAKE THE POP

The progestogen pill should be commenced on the first day of a woman's menstrual period with no extra precautions required. The POP is taken every day with no break. If your client needs to change to another progestogen pill, then the first pill of the new packet should be commenced the next day with no break, and no additional contraception will be required. Broad-spectrum antibiotics do not reduce the efficacy of the POP, so no extra precautions are required whilst taking them. The new DRSP POP is taken in a regimen of 24 daily active pills followed by 4 hormone-free placebo pills. The aim of the four hormone-free days is to try to establish a more predictable bleeding pattern (although the evidence suggests that this is not necessarily the case) whilst maintaining contraceptive effectiveness.

If the progestogen-only pill is commenced following a full-term pregnancy, then it should be started from day 21 after birth; no additional precautions are required. If your client has had a miscarriage or termination of pregnancy, then the POP should be commenced the same day or next day with no additional precautions required.

LOSS OF EFFICACY THROUGH DRUG INTERACTION

Enzyme-inducing drugs (see Table 7.3) reduce the efficacy of the POP, so another form of contraception should be discussed, e.g. the Depo-Provera injectable given at intervals of 12 weeks is preferable or condoms should be used whilst taking the drug and for 4 weeks after the enzyme-inducing drug has been ceased. HIV drugs can be checked on the website https://www.hiv-druginteractions.org.

Women who have taken ulipristal acetate emergency contraception (UPA-EC) should wait five days after taking UPA-EC before starting progestogen pills. They will need to use condoms reliably or abstain from sex during the five days before commencing the POP and then for a further two days after starting the LNG and NET POP, and for seven days with the DSG and DRSP POP (FSRH, August 2022a, amended July 2023).

Table 7.3 Enzyme-inducing drugs which reduce the efficacy of the POP. Up-to-date information on drug interactions can be found at https://bnf.nice.org.uk/interactions/

Drug type	Drug
Anticonvulsants	Carbamazepine
	Esilcarbamazepine
	Oxcarbazepine
	Fosphenytoin
	Phenytoin
	Perampanel
	Phenobarbital
	Primidone
	Topiramate
	Rufinamide

(Continued)

Table 7.3 Enzyme-inducing drugs which reduce the efficacy of the POP. Up-to-date information on drug interactions can be found at https://bnf.nice.org.uk/interactions/

Drug type	Drug
Antitubercle	Rifamycins, e.g. rifampicin, rifabutin
Antiretroviral – protease inhibitors	Ritonavir
	Ritonavir-boosted atazanavir
	Ritonavir-boosted tipranavir
	Ritonavir-boosted saquinavir
	Nelfinavir, darunavir, fosamprenavir, lopinavir
Antiretroviral – non-nucleoside reverse transcriptase inhibitors	Nevirapine
	Efavirenz
Other enzyme-inducing drugs	Modafinil
	Bosentan
	Aprepitant
Homeopathic	St John's Wort
Others	*Lamotrigine* (antiepileptic) and *griseofulvin* (antifungal). Contraceptive efficacy may be reduced by concurrent use of sugammadex

MISSED PILL RULES

If your client takes the desogestrel progestogen pill 12 or more hours late, she will need to take her pill as soon as she remembers and use extra precautions for two days of pills (Figure 7.1).

For all other traditional progestogen pills if she takes them three or more hours late, then she should be advised to take her pill when she remembers and use additional contraceptive precautions for the next two days of her pill (Figure 7.2).

If the new DRSP POP is taken more than 24 hours late, then she will need to use extra precautions for seven days. If these seven days fall into the four placebo pills, these will need to be omitted and enough active pills taken to equal seven pills (Figure 7.3).

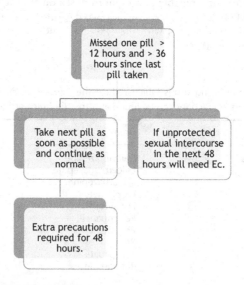

Figure 7.1 Missed desogestrel POP rules.

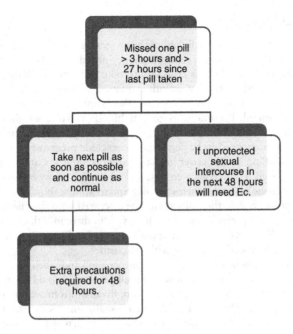

Figure 7.2 Missed traditional POP rules.

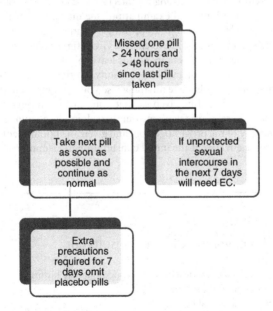

Figure 7.3 Missed drospirenone POP rules.

If a woman has severe diarrhoea or vomits within two hours of taking an LNG progestogen pill or three to four hours after taking DSG or DRSP progestogen pills, then extra precautions will be required for two days of pills with LNG progestogen pills and seven days with DSG and DRSP pills.

INITIAL CONSULTATION

When counselling a client initially about the progestogen-only pill, it is important to explain how this method prevents pregnancy and discuss its efficacy; this will help her to understand why it is necessary to take this type of pill on time. A full past and present medical history, including a family history, should be taken. If a client has a family history of heart disease, then appropriate screening for lipids should be performed. Routine screening of blood pressure, weight and height should be performed. Details about the last menstrual period are important, and a pregnancy test may need to be performed to exclude pregnancy.

Initial counselling should cover breast awareness, safer sex and cervical cytology history, as well as emergency contraception. If there is any evidence of cervical, uterine or pelvic infection, then screening and treatment should be undertaken. If a cervical smear is due, then this should be discussed with the client. It may be more appropriate to perform this at the next visit in three months' time. The progestogen pill will not protect against sexually transmitted infections or HIV – this issue should be discussed sensitively with the client.

You should discuss how to take the progestogen pill and when to use extra precautions. Side effects may be experienced initially, and you should warn your client that breast tenderness, bloatedness, depression, fluctuations in weight, nausea and irregular bleeding may be experienced. These usually improve with time, so it is important that she continues with the pill, as changing pill may perpetuate the problem. Your client may suffer from irregular bleeding, which may improve, but pathology should be excluded first. Screening for infection and cervical cytology should be performed along with a bimanual examination. She may also experience amenorrhoea, which may be due to the POP suppressing ovulation. However, if there is any likelihood of pregnancy, it should be excluded. Given time, your client may wish to discuss sexual anxieties, but sometimes clients leave this to the next visit when they know you better. Always give them the opportunity to bring up the subject by giving open-ended questions like, "Is there anything else you want to discuss?"

Up-to-date leaflets should be given so that your client can refer to them in an emergency along with relevant telephone numbers. Initially, a woman is prescribed three months' supply of the progestogen pill and given an appointment for this time.

The points to be covered at the initial consultation are summarised in Box 7.1.

Box 7.1

Points to be covered at initial consultation

- Full past and present medical history, including family history
- Record blood pressure, weight, height
- Details of last menstrual period
- Discuss efficacy of POP
- Teach how to take the pill and when to use extra precautions
- Discuss emergency contraception, safer sex, cervical cytology and breast awareness
- Discuss side effects
- Give appropriate leaflets and contact numbers

SUBSEQUENT VISITS

When a woman initially commences the POP, she will return for a follow-up visit in three months; if there are no problems, then she should be seen every six months after this. Discuss with her how she feels about the progestogen pill; has she taken it on time? Has she had any problems with her pill and what are they? Is she getting a regular menstrual cycle? If her menstrual cycle has been irregular, or she has experienced amenorrhoea, is this due to failure to take her pill on time, is there risk of pregnancy? A pregnancy test may need to be performed to exclude this.

Routine observations for blood pressure and weight should be performed. You may find that your client is more relaxed at this visit and may wish to discuss sexual problems or anxieties. This is also a good opportunity to discuss and perform cervical smears if due. You may need to revise how to take the progestogen pill, as clients have to take in a great deal of information at initial visits and may forget or be confused about missed pill rules.

If there are no problems, then a years' supply of the progestogen pill may be prescribed with a supply of condoms if required.

The points to be covered at subsequent visits are summarised in Box 7.2.

Box 7.2

Points to be covered at subsequent visits

- Update of medical and family history
- Basic observations – BP, weight, height
- Date of last menstrual period; has she had any problems with her pill?
- Is her cervical smear due?
- Is she breast aware?
- Do missed pill rules need revision?
- Safer sex – is she at risk?
- Has she got up-to-date leaflets on the POP and emergency contraception?
- Have relevant telephone numbers for advice been given?

POINTS TO BE COVERED AT SUBSEQUENT VISITS

SELF-ASSESSMENT QUESTIONS

Answers and discussion at the end of the chapter.

1 What problems would you envisage that a woman may encounter on the POP?
2 How would you solve these problems?
3 Which women are most suitable for the POP?
4 Which women are least suitable for the POP?

PROBLEMS ENCOUNTERED

- **NO MENSTRUAL PERIOD:**
  As long as pregnancy has been excluded, then you can reassure your client that her pill is working more effectively and preventing ovulation and periods.
- **IRREGULAR BLEEDING:**
  Check that your client is taking her pills correctly and not taking them late, which may put her at risk of pregnancy. Ask her to keep a diary of her bleeding pattern, so you can review this at the next visit. You should perform a pregnancy test and STI screen to eliminate the possibility she is pregnant or has a sexually transmitted infection, as these may cause irregular bleeding too. She may need to change to a different type of progestogen pill, or a different method.
- **COMPLAINTS OF NAUSEA:**
  Check that she is not taking her pill on an empty stomach. If the problem continues, change to a different progestogen.
- **BREAST TENDERNESS:**
  Examine breasts. Taking evening primrose oil can help to ease breast tenderness. Changing to a different progestogen may help.
- **PROBLEMS REMEMBERING PILLS:**
  If a woman is frequently forgetting to take her pill, then this will affect the efficacy of the progestogen pill and put her at risk of pregnancy. Check what time she is taking her pill; is there a more convenient time to take it? Can she set an alarm on her watch or computer diary or put a reminder on her mobile phone? What about carrying her packet around with her? Discuss with her how she feels about forgetting her pill. Would another method of contraception be more suitable?

SEXUALITY AND ANXIETIES

The progestogen pill may not always be a woman's first choice of contraception. She may have initially requested the combined pill but has a contraindication to it. This may affect compliance and increase dissatisfaction with the progestogen pill.

CASE HISTORY

A 24-year-old woman consults requesting to start the pill. She is aware of other methods but feels pills would suit her the best. The combined pill and the progestogen pill are discussed; the risks, disadvantages and advantages are fully covered. The client summarises the counselling by saying that the combined pill will have regular periods but has a risk of venous thromboembolism, whilst the desogestrel progestogen pill has the same effectiveness in preventing pregnancy and has less risks but irregular bleeding. She decides on this information to try the desogestrel progestogen pill as it has less risks and "put up with the irregular bleeding."

Many women hold the misconception that the progestogen pill is ineffective, because it was called the "mini pill," which may stop women from choosing it. However, it is a safe, reliable and effective method if taken consistently by the client.

Women who fail to take their pill on time may subconsciously wish to become pregnant but may not be ready to admit this to themselves. Given time and sensitive counselling, they may feel able to discuss this issue.

PROGESTOGEN-ONLY INJECTABLE (POI) CONTRACEPTION

Introduction and history

POI were initially a result of research following the war, when Dr Junkman found in 1953 that a long-acting injection was created if progestogen and alcohol were combined. In 1957, research began on the injectable Norigest, now known as Noristerat, which is licensed for short-term use in the UK, i.e. following administration of the rubella vaccine. In 1963 trials commenced on the injectable Depo-Provera, which was licensed in the UK for long-term use in 1984 when other methods were not suitable. Since 1990, it has been licensed as a first-choice method. Of the two injectables available, Depo-Provera is the most widely used. In 2015, Sayana Press was introduced to enable women to be able to self-administer subcutaneously medroxyprogesterone acetate (FSRH, 2015b).

Explanation of the method

Like the progestogen pill, POIs prevent pregnancy in several ways. They cause the cervical mucus to thicken, thus stopping sperm penetrability, render the endometrium unreceptive for implantation and reduce fallopian tube function. However, the main function of injectables in preventing pregnancy is suppression of ovulation.

Efficacy

The efficacy of POI is between 99% and 100% in preventing pregnancy; research has shown that POIs have a failure rate of 0.2% in the first year (December 2014, amended July 2023). Injectables are a highly effective form of contraception, as user failure rates are reduced. This is because women do not have to remember to take a pill, and there is no loss of efficacy caused through diarrhoea and vomiting.

Pharmacokinetics and pharmacodynamics

POIs are given parenterally and, as a result, absorbed directly into the blood stream and metabolised in the liver and excreted in faeces.

Disadvantages

- Irregular bleeding or spotting or amenorrhoea
- Delay in return of fertility of up to a year

- Depression
- Weight gain
- Galactorrhoea
- Once given cannot be withdrawn
- Small loss of bone mass density which usually is recovered once the injectable is stopped (FSRH, December 2014a, amended July 2023)
- Limited research between depot medroxyprogesterone acetate (DMPA) and breast cancer; the risk is likely to be small and reduce with time after stopping (FSRH, 2014a, amended July 2023)
- Small increased risk of meningioma in women using DMPA (FSRH, 2024c)

Advantages

- High efficacy
- Lasts 8–12 weeks depending on POI
- Reduction in dysmenorrhoea and menorrhagia, resulting in less anaemia
- Reduction in premenstrual symptoms
- Less pelvic inflammatory disease
- Possible reduction of endometriosis because of thickened cervical mucus
- Efficacy not reduced by diarrhoea, vomiting

UKMEC 4 unacceptable health risk – absolute contraindications

- Current breast cancer
- Pregnancy
- Allergy to a constituent
- Acute porphyrias
- Current osteoporosis, osteopenia

UKMEC 3 risks outweigh the benefits of using method – relative contraindications

- Multiple risk factors for cardiovascular disease
- History of breast cancer; the decision to commence any injectable should be made in consultation with oncology team (FSRH, 2016, amended 2019)
- Current history of ischaemic heart disease including cerebrovascular accident and transient ischaemic attack whilst taking progestogen methods needs to be reviewed
- High risk of osteoporosis
- Present liver disease, liver adenoma or cancer
- Severe decompensated cirrhosis
- Undiagnosed genital tract bleeding should be investigated

Range of method

There are three types of injectables (Table 7.4).

Table 7.4 Injectable contraceptives

Name	Progestogen	Dose	Administered
Depo-Provera Abbreviated to DMPA or IM DMPA	Medroxyprogesterone acetate	150 mg in 1 ml given IM	Every 12 weeks and 5 days
Sayana Press Abbreviated to SC DMPA	Medroxyprogesterone acetate	160 mg in 1 ml given subcutaneously	Every 13 weeks
Noristerat abbreviated to NET-EN	Norethisterone enanthate	200 mg in 1 ml given IM	Every 8 weeks

Decision of choice

Noristerat is licensed for short-term use only; this means no more than two consecutive injections. Noristerat (NET-EN) is usually used as a method following vasectomy or rubella administration where a highly effective method is required for a short period of time.

There are two types of injection preparations of DMPA intramuscular and subcutaneous. Depo-Provera, which contains DMPA 150mg in 1 ml is licensed for long-term use. Intramuscular DMPA should be given in the gluteal muscle. Subcutaneous (SC) DMPA injection Sayana Press (104 mg MPA in 0.65 ml) should be administered into the abdomen or anterior thigh, and there appear to have been more injection site reactions such as scarring and atrophy (December 2014, amended July 2023).

Progestogen injectables are suitable for most women, particularly those who forget their pills, and for women on the COC taking drugs where there is a loss of efficacy. However, there is a lack of information about long-term amenorrhoea, which is usually a result of this injection, and its implications.

In 1991, research (Cundy et al., 1991) suggested that women who are using long-term Depo-Provera may be partially oestrogen deficient; this may have an adverse effect on bone density and may give an increased risk of osteoporosis. However, Cundy et al. (1994) showed that this effect may be completely reversible once oestrogen levels have returned to normal following cessation of Depo-Provera. Gbolade (2002) states that loss of bone density in long-term users appears to be transient and reversible. Current advice by the FSRH based on available evidence says that POIs are associated with a small loss of bone mineral density which is reversible on discontinuation (December 2014, amended July 2023).

The FSRH and MHRA advise that women who are under the age of 18 whose peak bone mass may not have been reached may use progestogen injectables after all methods of contraception have been discussed and found not suitable (FSRH, December 2014a, amended July 2023). For women over the age of 50, the FSRH recommend that these women switch to an alternative method of contraception because of the theoretical risk of osteoporotic fracture in menopause. However, if these women do not wish to stop and have been assessed for the risks of osteoporosis and understand the potential risks, they may continue (December 2014, amended July 2023). They also recommend that all women who continue to use progestogen injectables should be reviewed every two years (December 2014, amended July 2023). Finally, women who have significant lifestyle or medical risk factors for osteoporosis should consider other methods of contraception (December 2014, amended July 2023). Risk factors for osteoporosis include personal history of fractures or anorexia nervosa and amenorrhoeic athletes, smoking and family history of osteoporosis in a first-degree relative, and use of steroids including oral steroids. Careful history taking to highlight these risks is important. Also, it is good practice to encourage women to maintain and build skeletal mass through diet, exercise and avoidance of smoking and alcohol.

There is a weak association between DMPA and breast cancer; the risk is likely to be small and reduce with time after stopping (December 2014, amended July 2023). There is no increased risk of cervical (International Family Planning Perspectives, 1992; WHO, 1992) or ovarian cancer with use of Depo-Provera; however, there is a protective effect for endometrial cancer (Pisake, 1994; December 2014, amended July 2023).

Studies show a small increased risk of meningioma in women using DMPA. Recent studies show that the average age of women in the study was 57.6, and the number of women exposed to medroxyprogesterone acetate was low (FSRH, 2024c). FSRH clinical effectiveness unit (CEU) advises that this is discussed with women, but there is no significant change to current practice (FSRH, 2024c).

When counselling women about POIs concerning the risk of osteoporosis and breast cancer, much of the research undertaken to date is limited. However, studies are consistent saying the risks are small.

Side effects

- Headaches
- Bloatedness
- Depression
- Weight gain
- Mood swings
- Irregular bleeding
- Amenorrhoea

How to give injectables

Ideally, Depo-Provera should be given within the first five days of a menstrual period; no additional contraception is required. After this, all injections should be given every 13 weeks (FSRH, 2014b, amended 2023), which is outside the product licence of 12 weeks.

Noristerat should be given on the first day of the menstrual period; no additional contraception required. After this, all injections should be given every eight weeks.

The intramuscular injections should be given deep intramuscularly into the upper outer quadrant of the buttock. The IM DMPA pre-filled syringe should be shaken well before being given. The NET-EN ampoule should be warmed to body temperature before being given. This will make it easier to draw up, as it is mixed with castor oil. Both injection sites should not be massaged after administration of the injectable, as this will reduce the efficacy. Subcutaneous DMPA should be shaken well before being given and administered into the abdomen or anterior thigh.

Following first trimester termination of pregnancy and miscarriage, the first injection is usually given within the first five days with no extra precautions required. Post-partum women should commence their first injectable day 21 following delivery (December 2014, amended July 2023).

101

Progestogen methods

Loss of efficacy through drug interaction

There is no loss of efficacy with Depo-Provera or Noristerat with broad-spectrum antibiotics and enzyme-inducing drugs; they should continue to be given at 12 weeks and 5 days for Depo-Provera. However, the FSRH say that subcutaneous and intramuscular Depo-Provera can be given every 13 weeks (which is outside the product licence) and 8 weeks for Noristerat (December 2014, amended July 2023).

SELF-ASSESSMENT QUESTIONS

Answers and discussion at the end of the chapter.

5   Who would you consider most suitable for using Depo-Provera as a method of contraception?
6   What would you do if a woman was beyond 12 weeks for her next Depo-Provera injection?
7   Name five issues that should be covered during counselling for women considering the Depo-Provera injection.

Initial consultation

Women who consult and who are interested in choosing Depo-Provera as a form of contraception should be counselled carefully, as this is a less easily reversed method. Counselling should cover the following areas to enable the woman to make an informed decision:

1   Once injected, it cannot be removed. It is important that women accept that once given, the injection cannot be withdrawn, so any unwanted side effects they experience, although usually short-lived, will continue until the injection expires at 12 weeks.
2   Efficacy and frequency of injections. Counselling should involve efficacy and how frequent injections need to be given. Occasionally, women have been under the impression that Depo-Provera is given every three months. This can be longer than 12 weeks, so it is important to talk about frequency of intervals in weeks. If a client is due a holiday, for example, then her injection can be given earlier.
3   Menstrual disturbances. Women should be warned that they may experience irregular bleeding initially with Depo-Provera or amenorrhoea within the first year. If warned beforehand, women usually find this acceptable.
4   Return of fertility. There can be a delay in the return of periods and fertility; however, most women will become pregnant within one year from stopping Depo-Provera. There is no evidence that Depo-Provera causes permanent infertility. If a woman is thinking of becoming pregnant in the near future, then another form of contraception may be more appropriate.

5 Weight gain and other minor side effects. There may be a small weight gain, so if women are aware of this, they will be able to monitor it, and it may be avoided.

6 Depression may be experienced by some women, although this may be due to outside factors.

7 Long-term use and the possible risk of osteoporosis are at present being researched. Clients often ask about the long-term effects of amenorrhoea, and as new information comes to light, they should be informed.

Women may wish to be given time before commencing injectables to think about their decision. Timing of the initial injection should be discussed along with alternative contraception. The first injection should be administered within the first five days of the cycle; otherwise, contraceptive precautions will be required for seven days. If there has been any unprotected sexual intercourse or if there is any concern over pregnancy, then a pregnancy test and bimanual examination if appropriate may need to be performed to exclude pregnancy.

Routine observations of weight, height and blood pressure should be done. A full medical of the woman and family history should be obtained. Previous contraceptive history should be discussed. If she has used a progestogen method previously it will give an impression of how she will experience the injectable. A cervical smear may need to be performed if due, although this may have to be deferred until the next injection if it is during her menses or if she prefers. Injectables do not protect against sexually transmitted diseases and HIV, so issues around safer sex may need to be discussed and approached with the woman.

Up-to-date literature about the injectable should be given, along with an appointment when the next injection will be due.

The points to be covered at the initial consultation are summarised in Box 7.3.

Box 7.3

Points to be covered at initial consultation

Full past and present medical history, including family history

- Record BP, weight, height
- Details of last menstrual period and any unprotected sexual intercourse
- Discuss efficacy of injectable
- Discuss intervals when injectables should be given
- Discuss emergency contraception, safer sex, cervical cytology and breast awareness
- Discuss side effects and issues around Depo-Provera (nos. 1–7)
- Give appropriate leaflets and contact numbers

Subsequent visits

Subsequent injections of Depo-Provera should be given every 12 weeks and Noristerat at 8-week intervals. Observations of blood pressure and weight should be performed. Regular weight checks can be useful, as often clients complain that their weight has increased, yet when weighed, there is no change.

At subsequent consultations, it is important to find out how your client is finding her injection. Is she experiencing any problems? How can these be alleviated? (see "Problems Encountered"). Most side effects of injectables are short-lived like BTB, so it is worth persevering with this method.

BOX 7.4

Points to be covered at subsequent visits

- Update of medical and family history
- Basic observations – BP, weight
- Has she had any problems, e.g. bleeding?
- Is her cervical smear due?
- Is she breast aware?
- Safer sex – is she at risk?
- Has she got up-to-date leaflets on the injectable?
- Have relevant telephone numbers for advice been given?
- It is important that your client knows when her next injection will be due and keeps a record of the date of her previous injection in case she needs to attend another nurse or doctor for her injection

PROBLEMS ENCOUNTERED

- IRREGULAR BLEEDING PATTERN:
  If a woman suffers irregular bleeding, she should be advised to return before her next injection is due so that it can be given earlier. If there is no improvement in the bleeding pattern, then she may be prescribed concurrent oestrogen either by the combined pill or if this is contraindicated by giving hormone replacement therapy.
  Most women who experience BTB find that this resolves usually by the fourth injection.
- COMPLAINTS OF INCREASED ACNE AND MOOD SWINGS:
  Some women may complain of increased acne or mood swings. This usually improves, but vitamin B6 and evening primrose oil may be beneficial. If there is no improvement in symptoms, then this should be discussed with the woman. She may wish to change method or treat the acne, for example, if she has a limited choice of contraception.
- CLIENTS ATTENDING LATE FOR INJECTIONS:
  Women who regularly attend late for their injections may need help with reminders. Some family planning clinics run domiciliary services for this reason or send their clients reminders. Try making your client's next appointment earlier at 12-week intervals.
  If your client is beyond 12 weeks and 5 days since her last injection of DMPA, then you may give it up to 14 weeks (or up to 10 weeks if NET-EN)

since the last injection with no extra precaution or emergency contraception is required.

If she is beyond 14 weeks and 1 day since her last DMPA or 10 weeks and 1 day since her last NET-EN, and there is no unprotected sexual intercourse, then you can give the DMPA or NET-EN with extra precautions required for 7 days and a pregnancy test is recommended in 21 days. If there is unprotected sex, and this is in the last 5 days, then emergency contraception via either levonorgestrel hormonal emergency contraception or a PCIUD will be required, and the injection may be given with extra precaution for 7 days. If ellaOne is given, then DMPA administration should be delayed and given in five days' time. Extra precautions will be required for 7 days after the injection is commenced and a pregnancy test performed in 21 days) (December 2014, amended July 2023).

If the last injection is more than 14 weeks and 1 day (or Noristerat 10 weeks and 1 day), and there is unprotected sex, and this is more than 5 days ago, then you are unable to give emergency contraception and you should advise alternative contraception or no sexual intercourse and perform a pregnancy test in 21 days. This is outside the drug license but is recommended practice by FSRH (December 2014, amended July 2023).

Sexuality and anxieties

Injectables are a highly effective form of contraception. They give a great deal of freedom to a woman, requiring a consultation only every 8–12 weeks. They allow women time to think and delay decisions about permanent methods of contraception. However, they are not a widely used method. Many women hold misconceptions about the injectable, which may also be held by professionals. Fears that the injection causes permanent infertility and foetal abnormality have been researched (Wilson, 1993). Although no evidence has been found to support these anxieties, they still remain. In the meantime, injectables are in many instances undervalued and many women are not even informed of the availability of this method.

Many women feel that having an injection which causes amenorrhoea is unnatural. There is concern about menstrual loss – "Where does it all go?" "Doesn't all the blood build up?" – which emphasises the need to explain clearly how the reproductive cycle works and how it is affected by the injectable. Women often forget that during pregnancy and whilst breast feeding, there is little or no bleeding, and this is natural. However, for some women, the experience of amenorrhoea can be too worrying. A period is the way women normally know whether they are pregnant or not and can be very reassuring.

PROGESTOGEN-ONLY IMPLANT

Introduction and history

In 1993, Norplant was the first implant to be approved for use in the UK as a contraceptive. Norplant was licensed for five years and is no longer manufactured.

Norplant received a great deal of adverse media attention after some women had problems with insertion and removal of the capsules, as a result, Implanon was launched. However, many women were very happy with Norplant. Implanon was a single capsule, reducing problems with insertion and removal. However, whilst Implanon was easier to fit and remove, the insertion procedure was slightly complicated; the manufacturers addressed this by developing Nexplanon in 2010. Nexplanon and Implanon are the same implants; however, the applicator and insertion technique for Nexplanon is more straightforward to ensure correct placement of the capsule, which is radiopaque. Nexplanon is now the only licensed implant in the UK.

Nexplanon should always be inserted by professionals who have undergone the designated training for this device, to avoid problems with incorrect insertion and as a result difficulties with removal.

A two-rod implant called Jadelle is available outside the UK, is licensed for five years and contains 75 mg of levonorgestrel.

Nexplanon

Nexplanon is a single rod which contains 68 mg of etonogestrel, a metabolite of the progestogen desogestrel, which is inserted subdermally and licensed for three years. The rod is 4 cm in length with a diameter of 2 mm and is provided with a sterile preloaded applicator and is radiopaque. Nexplanon prevents pregnancy by inhibiting ovulation, mucus and endometrial effect.

Efficacy

The implant's efficacy is less than 99.05% in the first year of use (FSRH, February 2021, amended July 2023).

There is no evidence to support a loss of efficacy by body weight or BMI with the implant (FSRH, February 2021, amended July 2023).

Disadvantages

- Requires a trained professional to insert and remove implants
- Irregular menstrual bleeding such as amenorrhoea or spotting
- Minor side effects such as headaches and acne
- Possible discomfort or infection at site

Advantages

- High efficacy
- Easily reversed
- Long-term contraception
- Free from oestrogen side effects
- Low user failure – once in place there is nothing to remember

UKMEC 4 unacceptable health risk – absolute contraindications

- Current breast cancer
- Pregnancy
- Allergy to components of implant

UKMEC 3 risks outweigh the benefits of using method – relative contraindications

- Undiagnosed genital tract bleeding
- Acute porphyria
- Current ischaemic heart disease, cardiovascular accident
- Severe decompensated liver cirrhosis
- Benign or malignant liver tumours
- Liver enzyme–inducing drugs
- Breast cancer in the last five years

Range of method

Nexplanon is the only implant available in the UK. It is 4 cm in length and 2 mm in diameter and is inserted with a disposable sterile applicator.

Side effects

- Irregular bleeding, amenorrhoea or frequent and prolonged bleeding
- Pain, itching or infection at insertion site
- Headaches
- Nausea
- Mood changes
- Weight changes
- Acne

Decision of choice

Women who are at risk of pregnancy or who have become pregnant because they have difficulty remembering to take a contraceptive pill or use another contraceptive method (user failure) may find Nexplanon a useful alternative. Women choosing an implant as their method of contraception should be counselled carefully about side effects, as this will influence their final decision. Implants are suitable for women who have completed their families or for women wishing to delay starting their family. Implants are reversible, and once removed, research has shown that 80% of women's menstrual cycle returned to normal or to their pre-trial pattern within three months (Edwards, 1999).

Counselling for Nexplanon

As Nexplanon involves a minor operation, it is important to counsel women fully so that they are able to make an informed decision. Women are also more likely to accept and continue with a method if they are aware of any side effects prior to the procedure.

You should discuss with your client the efficacy of Nexplanon and the procedure for insertion and removal. A full medical history should be taken along with family medical history. Side effects with Nexplanon are similar to any progestogen-only method, so if your client has previously tolerated a progestogen-only method well, then this will give you both a good indication on how she will feel with Nexplanon. If your client already suffers from symptoms such as headaches or acne, then Nexplanon may not improve these problems. However, many women, if warned, are prepared to accept continuing problems to be assured of a highly effective form of contraception.

Changes in menstrual pattern are the most frequently reported side effect of Nexplanon. Women may experience amenorrhoea, irregular menses or BTB. It is important to discuss the likelihood of amenorrhoea with Nexplanon, as this may cause anxiety. Many women find periods very reassuring, as they tell them that they are not pregnant, and as a result, amenorrhoea can cause great anxiety. Research on clinical experience with Norplant has shown that if women are given careful counselling on Norplant's effects on menstruation there is a higher continuation rate with this method (Mascarenhas et al., 1994), and the same could be said for all methods of contraception.

Following counselling, written up-to-date information should be given, so that your client is able to make an informed decision about Nexplanon.

It is important that your client uses contraception up to the time of Nexplanon insertion to exclude any possibility of pregnancy. Nexplanon should be preferably inserted on the first five days of your client's menstrual period, where no extra precautions will be required. If Nexplanon is inserted at any other time in the cycle, then pregnancy should be excluded first, and additional contraception should be used following insertion for seven days.

Following a termination of pregnancy, Nexplanon may be inserted immediately; if inserted later, then additional contraception will be required for seven days. After childbirth, Nexplanon may be inserted on day 21; if inserted later, then extra contraceptive precautions will be required for 7 days.

The areas to be covered at counselling are summarised in Box 7.5.

Box 7.5

Areas to be covered at counselling

- Full medical history
- Check blood pressure, weight and height
- Ensure client has contraceptive cover up to and after insertion if needed
- Take details of last menstrual period; exclude pregnancy if relevant
- Discuss how Nexplanon works and its efficacy
- Discuss insertion and removal procedure
- Discuss side effects
- Give literature on Nexplanon
- Organise date for insertion

Drugs which reduce the efficacy of Nexplanon

The enzyme-inducing drugs that reduce the efficacy of Nexplanon are listed in Table 7.5

Progestogen receptor modulators such as ulipristal acetate may potentially reduce the efficacy of the implant. As a result, Implanon cannot be quick started for five days after taking ulipristal acetate, and extra precautions will be required for seven days after insertion (FSRH, February 2021, amended July 2023). Additional contraception is required with Nexplanon if drugs are liver enzyme–inducing; additional barrier contraception will be required whilst taking the drugs and for 28 days after their cessation (FSRH, February 2021, amended July 2023) or alternatively a client can be given the injectable contraceptive Depo-Provera with no extra precautions required.

Nexplanon insertion

Nexplanon is inserted with a sterile technique under local anaesthetic into the inner aspect of the upper arm of the non-dominant arm avoiding the sulcus between the biceps and triceps. Insertion of Nexplanon is performed with a specially designed applicator. Nexplanon should be inserted at the inner side of the upper arm about 8–10 cm above the medial epicondyle of the humerus along the sulcal line and then 3–5 cm posteriorly perpendicular to the sulcal line (FSRH, February 2021, amended July 2023).

Table 7.5 Enzyme-inducing drugs that reduce the efficacy of Nexplanon. Up-to-date information on drug interactions can be found at https://bnf.nice.org.uk/interactions/

Drug type	Drug
Anticonvulsants	Carbamazepine
	Esilcarbamazepine
	Oxcarbazepine
	Fosphenytoin
	Phenytoin
	Perampanel
	Phenobarbital
	Primidone
	Topiramate
	Rufinamide
Antitubercle	Rifamycins, e.g. rifampicin, rifabutin
Antiretroviral – protease inhibitors	Ritonavir
	Ritonavir-boosted atazanavir
	Ritonavir-boosted tipranavir
	Ritonavir-boosted saquinavir
	Nelfinavir, darunavir, fosamprenavir, lopinavir
Antiretroviral – non-nucleoside reverse transcriptase inhibitors	Nevirapine
	Efavirenz
Other enzyme-inducing drugs	Modafinil
	Bosentan
	Aprepitant
Homeopathic	St John's Wort
Others	*Lamotrigine* (antiepileptic) and *griseofulvin* (antifungal) contraceptive efficacy may be reduced by concurrent use of sugammadex

The insertion site should be marked and cleaned with disinfectant, and local anaesthetic given. The skin should be stretched and the tip of the implant applicator inserted into the site at a slight angle of 30°. The capsule is held inside the applicator at the tip. Release the skin and lower the applicator to a horizontal position; lift the skin with the tip of the needle but keep the needle in the subdermal connective tissue. Whilst lifting the skin gently, insert the needle to its full length without using force. The purple slider is unlocked by pushing it slightly down, and the slider is moved back until it stops; this releases the implant subdermally and locks the needle in the applicator. The applicator is removed, and the implant should be palpated. A dry dressing and pressure bandage are applied, which can be removed in 24 hours. The insertion procedure takes 15 minutes. Batch number and expiry date of the implant should be recorded in the clients notes.

Women should be able to feel the capsules once *in situ* if they wish to touch the site for reassurance, but they will not be visible unless the woman is very thin. A user card should be given to the client which includes the batch number, date of insertion, the arm where the implant is inserted, name of the inserter and hospital and the intended date of removal.

ACTIVITY

Watch the YouTube video of an implant insertion and removal produced by Worcestershire Health and Care NHS Trust at https://www.youtube.com/watch?v=opnXt3m2Nno.

The College of Sexual and Reproductive Healthcare (CoSRH) has a training scheme for the fitting and removal of implants. A letter of competence in subdermal contraceptive implants for Faculty members is for five years from issue, and there is a regional network of advisors.

Subsequent visits

You should advise your client to return if she has any problems. She should be advised when to return for removal and how to palpate the implant.

Nexplanon removal

Removal of Nexplanon should only be performed by a professional who is familiar with the removal technique. Removal of the implants is performed under sterile technique with local anaesthetic. The location of the implant should be indicated on the user card, and the location palpated and the marked at the distal end. A non-palpable implant should be located by ultrasound or magnetic resonance imaging and removed with the aid of ultrasound.

For removal, the area should be cleaned, and local anaesthetic inserted under the implant. An incision of 2 mm in length is made longitudinally; the implant should be pushed towards the incision until the tip is visible and then be grasped with forceps and removed. The incision site should have a Steri-Strip applied and sterile dressing and pressure bandage applied.

If your client wishes to continue using Nexplanon as a method of contraception, then a new implant may be inserted in a parallel plane from those removed through the same incision. However, if she is discontinuing with this method, alternative contraception is required once the capsule is removed.

SELF-ASSESSMENT QUESTIONS

Answers and discussion at the end of the chapter.

8 Who do you think is suitable for Nexplanon?
9 What would you do if your client complained of amenorrhoea?
10 How long can Nexplanon remain *in situ*, and when does fertility return?
11 When would you advise your client that she would need to commence alternative contraception following removal?

PROBLEMS ENCOUNTERED

■ IRREGULAR BLEEDING:
Research has shown that one of the main reasons for discontinuing Nexplanon is due to complaints of irregular bleeding.

Women who experience persistent irregular bleeding should be screened for sexually transmitted infections, cervical cytology and pregnancy to exclude the possibility of pregnancy or chlamydia/gonorrhoea infection firstly. If these are negative and the combined pill is not contraindicated, then a three-month supply of a levonorgestrel-containing pill (second generation) can be given, which can be taken continuously or in cyclical regimen. The combined pill is unlicensed for this use, but this practice is endorsed by FSRH (February 2021, amended July 2023; FSRH, 2015e). If the combined pill is contraindicated, then mefenamic acid can be prescribed 500 mg up to three times a day for five days. These regimens may have a beneficial effect, but there is limited data on their success; however, women should be warned that bleeding may return. Women who experience amenorrhoea with Nexplanon may be alarmed at the loss of their menses if they are not warned prior to insertion. Explaining how Nexplanon prevents pregnancy and why amenorrhoea occurs can help prevent anxiety.

■ PREMENSTRUAL-LIKE SYMPTOMS:
Women may find that taking evening primrose oil or vitamin B6 will help relieve premenstrual-like symptoms, such as irritability and mood swings.

Case history

A 26-year-old woman named Jan has two children, aged two and three. She has had a miscarriage prior to having her children and three months ago a termination of pregnancy. Jan has requested a sterilisation but her present relationship is a new one, and it has been suggested that she wait a little longer. She is 5'3" (159 cm) and weighs 15 stone 2 lb (96 kg) and was taking the combined pill but has changed to the progestogen pill, which she finds difficult to remember to take on time. Jan has always suffered from painful, heavy periods, and all her pregnancies have been unplanned.

The combined pill is contraindicated in this situation because the BMI is 38 kg m^2. She is unsuitable for an intrauterine contraceptive device (CU-IUD) because of her dysmenorrhoea and menorrhagia.

Three long-term methods of contraception are discussed with Jan: the injectable Depo-Provera, the implant Nexplanon and the levonorgestrel intrauterine device (LNG-IUD). Jan is reluctant to have the LNG-IUD because she does not like the idea of the insertion. She feels that she may not remember to attend for injections every 11–12 weeks, leaving Nexplanon as the method of choice. Although she is not keen on the insertion of Nexplanon, she prefers this over a LNG-IUD insertion and decides to go ahead with this as a method of contraception. Nexplanon is a safe contraceptive option for women who are overweight, and evidence suggests that efficacy is not reduced by body weight or BMI (FSRH, February 2021, amended July 2023).

Sexuality and anxieties

Women who choose Nexplanon find its high efficacy and lack of user compliance important advantages. They may be unable to use other methods because of medical contraindications or wish to use a method that is long term without making the final permanent decision of sterilisation.

ANSWERS TO SELF-ASSESSMENT QUESTIONS OF POP

1   What problems would you envisage that a woman may encounter on the POP?
    Women may complain of premenstrual-like symptom such as breast tenderness, nausea, irregular bleeding or amenorrhoea. They may find it difficult to remember when to take their pill, and if they have taken the combined pill previously, they may dislike the lack of warning of their menstrual cycle.
2   How would you solve these problems?
    Nausea can be solved by always taking your pill after food. Premenstrual-like symptoms may be reduced by trying evening primrose oil and vitamin B6. If there is no improvement, then changing to a different POP may help.
    Problems with irregular bleeding and amenorrhoea should be discussed. Often, if women are fully counselled into how the POP works in preventing pregnancy, they are more ready to accept any problems. Check that they are taking their pills correctly: Do they understand the importance of this in relation to efficacy?
3   Which women are most suitable for the POP?
    Women who are most suitable to take the POP are those who are breast feeding and who are older. It is also suitable for diabetic women, or for women undergoing surgery or women who suffer migraines or have had a venous thromboembolism or who smoke – all of whom are unable to take the

combined pill. There are in fact very few women who are not suitable for this method!

4 Which women are least suitable for the POP?

Women who are less suitable to take the POP are women who are unreliable at taking pills or who find the irregular bleeding a problem. It is not suitable for women who are taking liver enzyme–inducing drugs where there will be loss of efficacy. It is not suitable for women who are pregnant, and women who have had an ectopic pregnancy or who have been hospitalised with functional ovarian cysts should be given desogestrel progestogen pill, as this will inhibit ovulation and reduce the risk of functional ovarian cysts and ectopic pregnancy.

Any woman who has experienced a problem with the combined pill which may not be related to the oestrogen content of the COC or has had a malignancy of the breast should not be given the POP. Women who have liver disease, arterial disease or any drug which may reduce the efficacy of the POP.

Table 7.4 shows drugs which affect the efficacy of the POP outlined here. Enzyme-inducing drugs reduce the efficacy of the POP by the induction of liver enzymes, which increase the metabolism of the progestogen pill.

ANSWERS TO SELF-ASSESSMENT QUESTIONS FOR INJECTABLES

5 Who would you consider most suitable for using Depo-Provera as a method of contraception?

Women who are most suitable for Depo-Provera are as follows:

- Women who do not want to become pregnant but are not yet ready to choose sterilisation or do not wish to become pregnant in the foreseeable future
- Women who are having treatment with liver enzyme–inducing drugs, e.g. rifampicin for tuberculosis
- Women who are unable to take the combined pill
- Young women who want a highly effective form of contraception but either do not want to take the COC or have an absolute contraindication to it or find it difficult to remember to take it

6 What would you do if a woman was beyond 12 weeks for her next Depo-Provera injection?

If your client has gone beyond 12 weeks and 5 days, then you can give the next injection if it is within 14 weeks with no need for emergency contraception or extra precautions required. If beyond 14 weeks and 1 day, look at the "Problems Encountered" section.

7 Name five issues that should be covered during counselling for women considering the Depo-Provera injection.

Five issues that should be discussed during counselling include the following:

1 Efficacy
2 Delay in return of fertility
3 Amenorrhoea and irregular bleeding pattern
4 Once given the injection, it cannot be withdrawn
5 Side effects, e.g. weight gain, depression and long-term effects of injectables which are uncertain, like research into osteoporosis

ANSWERS TO SELF-ASSESSMENT QUESTIONS FOR IMPLANTS

8 Who do you think is suitable for Nexplanon?
Women who are most suitable for Nexplanon are those who have completed their families or who do not wish to have children in the near future. Nexplanon is also suitable for women who may be unable to use another method because they have a contraindication to them, e.g. the combined pill and focal migraines or menorrhagia and the IUCD.
9 What would you do if your client complained of amenorrhoea?
It is important to exclude pregnancy first. Once this has been excluded, then you should discuss with your client why amenorrhoea occurs with Nexplanon.
10 How long can Nexplanon remain *in situ*, and when does fertility return?
Nexplanon can remain *in situ* for three years. Fertility returns immediately after the capsules are removed.
11 When would you advise your client that she would need to commence alternative contraception following removal?
Another method of contraception should be used immediately after Nexplanon is removed.

8 INTRAUTERINE CONTRACEPTION

INTRODUCTION

The term "intrauterine contraception" (IUC) encompasses copper intrauterine devices (Cu-IUD) and levonorgestrel intrauterine devices (LNG-IUD), previously referred to as the LNG-IUD (intrauterine system). Both of these types of devices are long acting and reversible.

Copper IUDs have copper wound around the stem and or the arms of the device and have a copper surface area of ≥ 300 mm^2, this gives Cu-IUDs their high efficacy. The LNG-IUDs does not have any copper on the device but instead contains progestogen in the form of levonorgestrel in its stem. There are three different doses available of levonorgestrel in LNG- IUDs: 52, 19.5 or 13.5 mg.

THE COPPER IUD

The Cu-IUD is often referred to as the "coil" and has fewer side effects, has increased efficacy and lasts up to ten years; it is the only intrauterine device which can be inserted as emergency contraception.

EXPLANATION OF METHOD

A Copper intrauterine device (Cu-IUD) is inserted through the cervical canal and sits in the uterus. It has threads which hang down into the vagina, which a woman can check to make sure that the device is correctly positioned. It prevents pregnancy by impairing the viability of the sperm and ovum through the alteration of the fallopian tube and uterine fluids; there is a foreign body reaction with an increase in leucocytes. This reduces the chances of the ovum and sperm from meeting and impedes fertilisation. The copper in Cu-IUD is believed to be toxic to sperm and ovum.

EFFICACY

Cu-IUDs are highly effective, with an efficacy of 99.4%–99.8% in the first year of use, and they are not affected by enzyme-inducing drugs or weight/body mass index (FSRH, 2023a).

DOI: 10.4324/9781003484424-9

TIMING OF INSERTION OF CU-IUD

A Cu-IUD can be fitted at any time in the cycle if pregnancy can be excluded (FSRH, 2023a). To exclude pregnancy, clinicians should be certain the no sexual intercourse has occurred or that the person has used reliable contraception consistently, or they are within the first five days of the onset of a normal (natural) menstrual period. Women who are post-partum can have an IUD fitted within 48 hours after childbirth or from 21 days post-partum (non-breastfeeding individuals; FSRH, 2023a).

However, it may be difficult to exclude pregnancy; then a Cu-IUD can be fitted as emergency contraception if either of the following occurs:

1 It is within five days after the first episode of unprotected sexual intercourse in that cycle.
2 It is within five days of the earliest expected date of ovulation (FSRH, 2023a).

DISADVANTAGES

■ Menorrhagia
■ Dysmenorrhoea
■ Slightly increased risk of ectopic pregnancy if there is an IUD failure
■ Increased risk of pelvic infection (see p. 118)
■ Expulsion of the IUD
■ Perforation of the uterus, bowel and bladder
■ Malposition of the IUD
■ Pregnancy caused by expulsion, perforation or malposition

ADVANTAGES

■ Effective immediately
■ No drug interactions
■ Reversible and highly effective
■ Not related to sexual intercourse

UKMEC 4 unacceptable health risk – absolute contraindications

■ Pregnancy
■ Post-partum sepsis
■ Post-abortion sepsis
■ Unexplained vaginal bleeding should be investigated before insertion
■ Gestational trophoblastic disease with persistent elevated beta HCG levels or malignant disease
■ Awaiting treatment for cervical cancer, endometrial cancer
■ Undiagnosed genital tract bleeding (once the cause has been diagnosed and treated, an IUD may be inserted)
■ Pelvic or vaginal infection such as symptomatic chlamydia or gonorrhoea (once treated, an IUD may be fitted)

- Known pelvic tuberculosis
- Endometrial cancer
- Allergy to components of IUD, e.g. copper
- Wilson's disease

UKMEC 3 risks outweigh the benefits of using method – relative contraindications

- Less than four weeks post-partum
- Abnormalities of the uterus, e.g. bicornuate uterus, fibroids
- Inherited bleeding disorders (haematologist advice should be sought about inserting the device)
- Dysmenorrhoea and/or menorrhagia
- Organ transplant (for initiation)
- Known long QT syndrome (for initiation)
- HIV is classified as UKMEC3 for insertion if CD4 count < 200 and UKMEC2 for continuation. This is because of reduced immune system caused by the HIV virus and, as a result, an increased risk of infection

RANGE OF METHOD

There are 18 intrauterine devices available in the UK. Three different IUDs are shown in Figure 8.1, and Table 8.1 lists all 18 together with details of their life span and construction.

SIDE EFFECTS

- Menorrhagia
- Dysmenorrhoea

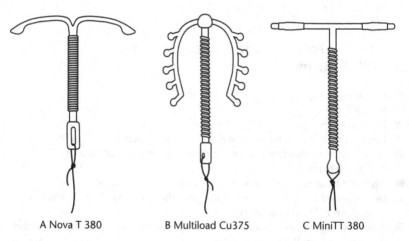

| A Nova T 380 | B Multiload Cu375 | C MiniTT 380 |

Figure 8.1 Three IUDs.

Table 8.1 Names and details of lifespan and construction of intrauterine devices

Device	Lifespan	Construction
Multiload Cu375	5 years	Vertical stem 3.5 cm in length; 375 mm^2 of copper wound around
Multi-Safe 375	5 years	375 mm^2 of copper wound around stem
Copper T380 A	10 years	380 mm^2 wound around stem and copper collar around each distal portion of each arm
Flexi-T 300	5 years	300 mm^2 of copper wound around stem
Flexi-T 380	5 years	380 mm^2 of copper wound around stem
Nova T 380	5 years	380 mm^2 of copper wire with silver core wound around stem
Load 375	5 years	U-shaped with 375 mm^2 copper wire wound stem
Mini TT380 Slimline	5 years	380 mm^2 wound around stem and copper collar around each distal portion of each arm
Neo-safe T 380	5 years	T-shaped with 380 mm^2 copper wire wound stem
T Safe 380A Quick Load	10 years	380 mm^2 wound around stem and copper collar around each distal portion of each arm
TT380 Slimline	10 years	380 mm^2 wound around stem and copper collar around each distal portion of each arm
Novaplus T 380 Cu	5 years	380mm^2 of copper wound around stem
Novaplus T 380 AG	5 years	380 mm^2 of copper wound around stem
UT 380 Standard	5 years	380 mm^2 of copper wound around the stem
UT 380 Short	5 years	380 mm^2 of copper wound around the stem
GyneFix	5 years	Frameless IUD with six copper tubes each 5 mm in length and 2.2 mm in diameter with total 330 mm^2 of copper wound around stem and arms
Ancora 375 cu	5 years	375 mm^2 of copper wound around the stem
IUB Ballerine Midi	5 years	300 mm of copper

DECISION OF CHOICE

The decision of which Cu-IUD to insert will depend on the woman and the size of her uterus. The Flexi T300, the Flexi-T 300 and Mini TT380 Slimline are suitable for a uterus of 5 cm in length; the Flexi-T 380 is suitable for a uterine length of over 6 cm, a Load 375 suitable for uterine length of over 7 cm; and the Multiload Cu375 and the Multi-safe 375 are suitable for uterine length of 6–9 cm. The Novaplus T 380, T Safe 380A Quickload, Neo-Safe T380, Copper T380A, UT380 standard and TT380 Slimline are suitable for a uterine length of over 6.5–9 cm.

Complications are most likely to occur at the insertion of an IUD. Perforation of the uterus, vasovagal shock, expulsion of the IUD, pelvic infection, pain and bleeding may occur following insertion or in the first year of use. The T Cu380A and TCU380 Slimline are the current favoured 380 IUDs available in the UK for insertions, offering the highest efficacy and licensed for ten years, which means that the risks associated with insertion are decreased, as it does not require frequent changing. High-copper devices with at least 380 mm of copper and copper bands on the transverse arms have the highest contraceptive efficacy (FSRH, 2023a).

Research suggests that frameless intrauterine devices such as GyneFix have a higher failure rate in comparison to framed Cu-IUDs (FSRH, 2023). Another type of frameless device is the intrauterine ball (IUB) a copper intrauterine device consisting of copper beads. Once the IUB is released from the insertion tube into the uterus, the IUB coils into a spherical shape measuring 15 mm. A blue thread is attached at one end to aid detection and removal. Currently, there is limited data on this method, but one small study showed a high expulsion rate of 27%; the FSRH Clinical Effectiveness Unit will continue to monitor evidence (FSRH, 2019f).

If a woman wishes to have an IUD fitted, then the most suitable IUD will be one which has a long licence and high efficacy, resulting in lower risk of pelvic infection, expulsion and perforation. However, the IUD inserted will also depend on the size and shape of a woman's uterus, and the inserter will take into consideration all these factors when choosing which device to fit.

IUD COUNSELLING

When counselling a woman about an intrauterine device, you should take a full past and present medical history, which will help to exclude any absolute contraindications. Your discussion of the efficacy and risks of an IUD should include the following points.

1 Clients should be aware that their periods may be heavier and more painful. Menstrual periods may improve within a few months after insertion. If they are already painful and heavy, another form of contraception may be more suitable like the levonorgestrel LNG-IUD.

2 Research on the risk of pelvic infection is limited. Hubacher et al. (2013) have discussed the barriers within researching this area. These include the difficulty ascertaining the timing of the exposure to the infection, the lack of an appropriate comparison group and inaccuracies over diagnosing pelvic infection (Hubacher et al., 2013; FSRH, 2015d). However, the risk of pelvic infection is considered to be low and less than 1% but is the highest in the first three weeks following insertion (FSRH, 2023).

An IUD will not protect any woman against STIs and HIV, so these issues need to be approached with her. If your client is not in a permanent relationship and wishes to have an IUD inserted, then her risk to exposure to STIs may be higher, and this should be discussed along with safer sex.

Women who are asymptomatic should be screened for sexually transmitted infections but do not have to wait for the results before the IUD is inserted (FSRH, 2023a). If a woman is having a post-coital IUD inserted, then prophylactic antibiotics are not necessary, and screening for chlamydia and gonorrhoea should be performed at insertion (FSRH, 2023a). However, any woman who is experiencing symptoms of a STI, e.g. dyspareunia (painful sexual intercourse), offensive discharge or on vaginal examination is found to have cervical excitation, pelvic pain or cervicitis, should have a full screening for STIs performed and ideally the IUD delayed until the results are confirmed.

You should encourage your client to attend earlier following an IUD insertion if she experiences any signs of vaginal infection, such as abdominal pain, along with pyrexia, so that full infection screening can be performed and antibiotics given early to prevent pelvic infection.

3 You should discuss with your client the risk of expulsion of the IUD, which occurs in approximately 1 in 20 women (FSRH, 2023a). This is most likely to occur in the first three months following insertion. Ideally, a follow-up

consultation is offered four to six weeks after insertion to ensure that there are no problems with the device. All women should be taught to check their IUD threads every month after menstruation. If they can feel the end of the IUD, which will feel like the end of a matchstick, they should be advised to use alternative contraception and return to see you.

4 There is a rare risk that during insertion, the IUD may perforate the uterus or cervix; the risk of this happening is 1–2 per 1,000 insertions and is six times higher in breast feeding women (FSRH, 2023a). If your client experiences low abdominal pain which continues following insertion with no improvement, she should be advised to see a doctor.

5 Efficacy should be discussed with women, as no form of contraception is 100% effective against pregnancy. If an IUD fails, then there is a risk that a pregnancy may be an ectopic pregnancy, so you should advise women to return early so this can be excluded. If she experiences low abdominal pain which is persistent and either missed or scanty periods, she should seek help immediately.

An IUD is usually inserted at the end of a menstrual period, as the cervix is slightly opened at this time, making insertion easier. An IUD may be inserted up to five days after the earliest calculated day of ovulation as post-coital contraception. Following delivery of a baby, a woman can have an IUD fitted six weeks postnatally. After a miscarriage or a termination of pregnancy, an IUD may be inserted immediately if the pregnancy was less than 12 weeks.

It is a good idea to encourage women to eat prior to an IUD insertion, as they will then be less likely to feel faint following insertion. Many women allow themselves little or no time to recover from insertion. Following insertion, they may experience cramp-like period pains, and it can be helpful to warn them to allow more time for themselves and perhaps organise for someone else to pick up their children or leave work earlier that day.

The areas to be covered at counselling are summarised in Box 8.1.

Box 8.1

Areas to be covered during counselling

- Full medical history
- Check blood pressure, weight and height
- Ensure client has contraceptive cover up to insertion
- Take details of last menstrual period; exclude pregnancy if relevant
- Discuss how an IUD works and its efficacy
- Discuss insertion and removal procedure
- Discuss side effects, e.g. heavy painful periods
- Discuss risks of insertion – expulsion, perforation, pregnancy and ectopic pregnancy
- Perform bimanual examination to exclude contraindications and take chlamydia and gonorrhoea swab
- Discuss risk of infection and safer sex
- Give literature on IUD

INSERTION PROCEDURE

Prior to insertion the chlamydia and gonorrhoea result should be checked, information about the last menstrual period obtained to exclude an already present pregnancy and a pregnancy test performed if required. Research (Guillebaud and Bounds, 1983) has shown that if mefenamic acid 500 mg is given orally prior to insertion, there is a reduction in pain following insertion of an IUD. Women should empty their bladders prior to insertion, as this will make it easier for the inserter to feel the uterus abdominally, and it will be more comfortable for the woman. The use of prophylactic antibiotics with immunocompromised women should be assessed individually and discussed with the woman's consultant (FSRH, 2023a).

During the IUD insertion procedure, your client may like to have someone to hold her hand and comfort her; this may be you or a friend or partner. Prior to insertion, a bimanual examination will be performed by the inserter to ascertain the size, position and direction of the uterus, and to check that there is no tenderness.

The skill and expertise of the inserter will help reduce any problems and side effects. However, if a woman would like to have local anaesthetic to reduce pain or has had problems with an IUD in the past, then it can be given with lignocaine gel or a paracervical block using lignocaine. She may need to be referred to a hospital clinic which specialises in difficult insertions and removals.

Insertion of an IUD is performed by a "non-touch technique," so a clean pair of gloves should be used following bimanual examination. A sterile speculum is inserted into the vagina, and the cervix is located; this is cleaned with sterile cotton wool and antiseptic solution. A uterine sound is inserted into the uterus via the cervical canal to measure the length, direction and patency of the uterus. This may cause cramp-like period pains which should diminish when the uterine sound is removed. The cervix may be stabilised by Allis forceps or a tenaculum so that the IUD may be inserted more easily; these may cause some discomfort, as the cervix is very sensitive. Next, the IUD is inserted through the cervical canal into the uterus. The threads of the IUD are shortened once it is in position and are tucked up behind the cervix. If there are any problems with an insertion, then your client should be referred to a specialist in IUDs. Following insertion, you should encourage your client to lie down and rest. Analgesia may be required for period pains. Sanitary towels should be used initially to reduce the risk of infection and because tampons may catch on the IUD threads which have not yet softened. Tampons may be used with the next menstrual period. Your client may experience bleeding initially. This is a good time to remind her of any initial problems and when to return — for example, if she experiences a change in her normal vaginal discharge or persistent abdominal pain. You should teach your client how to check her IUD threads and encourage her to perform this after each menstrual period. It is helpful to show your client a picture of the type of IUD she has fitted and how long it should remain in situ. Up-to-date written information should be given along with relevant telephone numbers of where to get help if needed. The IUD is effective immediately, so no additional contraception is required. An IUD procedure usually takes ten minutes.

VASOVAGAL AND ANAPHYLAXIS ATTACKS

Vasovagal and anaphylaxis attacks are usually rare; however, it is important to have emergency equipment and clear guidelines available for such events. Your client may feel sweaty and complain of feeling faint or sick. She may look pale, and her pulse may be slower. If the IUD insertion procedure is still in progress, then it should be stopped, and the woman should be laid in supine position with her head lowered and feet raised. If bradycardia persists, then slow intravenous atropine 500 to 600 mcg may be required by a suitably trained professional. If the woman has difficulty breathing and there is loss of consciousness and absence of a carotid pulse, her airway should be maintained by using pocket mask and emergency services phoned and help summoned. She should be laid in the left lateral position, and if there is no central pulse then 1mg adrenaline (= 10 ml 1:10 000) as a prefilled syringe may be given by deep intramuscular injection. If there is no improvement, this may be repeated at 5-minute intervals (Joint Formulary Committee, 2023). If required, cardiopulmonary resuscitation should be commenced. The woman should never be left unattended at any time (FSRH, 2023a).

POST-FITTING

After fitting an IUD, it is important to encourage women to return earlier than the 4- to 6-week appointment if they suffer from any signs of infection, as the first 20 days after fitting are the highest infection time. If a client suffers from low abdominal pain or pyrexia, then they should return early. It is good practice to encourage women to abstain from sexual intercourse for 48 hours so that the cervical mucus has returned to normal, helping to give some protection against transcending infection.

SUBSEQUENT VISITS

Ideally you should see your client four to six weeks post IUD insertion to examine and discuss any problems she may have. Details of the last menstrual period should be taken, along with any problems she has experienced. You should ask about any pain or difficulties having sexual intercourse; can her partner feel the IUD threads? Has she been able to check her threads herself? This information will help you when you examine your client, as it will give you signs for infection, and you will be able to re-teach your client how to check her threads if she is unable to do so. Your client should be examined with a speculum first so that the IUD threads may be observed. If the IUD threads appear too long, they may be shortened. If a cervical smear is required, then it may be taken at this time. After the speculum examination, a bimanual examination should be performed. If the tip of the IUD can be felt in the cervical os, which might not have been seen on speculum examination, then the IUD is too low in the uterine cavity and will need to be removed and a new device fitted. The cervix should be checked for cervical excitation by moving it gently from side to side. If pain is experienced whilst this is performed, it may indicate infection or an ectopic pregnancy. If any signs of vaginal or pelvic infection are observed, then you should refer your client to a genitourinary medicine clinic for full infection screening if unavailable on site.

REMOVAL PROCEDURE

An IUD may be removed if there is no unprotected sexual intercourse in the last seven days. Alternative contraception should be commenced at least seven days prior to removal. If an IUD is being changed and a problem arises which prevents insertion of a new device, then emergency hormonal contraception may be indicated for sexual intercourse prior to removal of the old device.

An IUD is removed by inserting a speculum into the vagina and locating the cervix, from which the IUD threads should be visible. Spencer Wells forceps are applied to the IUD threads and gentle traction is applied. The IUD should slowly descend into the vagina. If this does not happen, then it may be because the IUD has become embedded in the uterus, and you should refer your client to a specialist doctor experienced in difficult removals.

It is usually advised that IUDs are removed one year after the last menstrual period in menopausal women over the age of 50 and two years after the last menstrual period in women under the age of 50, because there is concern that an IUD may cause pyometra (pus in the uterus) (CSAC, 1993; FSRH, 2023a).

SELF-ASSESSMENT QUESTIONS

Answers and discussion at the end of the chapter.

1 Your client, who has IUD in situ, is concerned that her menstrual period is two weeks late. What would you do?
2 A 45-year-old woman attends for her IUD to be changed. It was inserted five years ago and is a Novaplus T 380. What would you do in this situation, and what further information do you need to know?
3 A 35-year-old woman consults complaining of dyspareunia for two months. She is in a permanent relationship and has had an IUD in situ for two years with no previous problems. What would you do in this situation?

PROBLEMS ENCOUNTERED

■ LOST THREADS:

If you or your client are unable to feel the IUD threads, this may indicate that the IUD has been expelled or that the IUD has moved within the uterus or perforated the uterus, taking the threads with it. You should advise your client to use alternative contraception, as she may be at risk of pregnancy. However, she may already be pregnant, and a pregnancy test should be performed to exclude this, along with details of her last menstrual period and any signs of pregnancy which may be experienced. Extrauterine pregnancy should be excluded first by ultrasound scan. If your client has an intrauterine pregnancy and wishes to continue with the pregnancy, the IUD may be left in situ if it is too difficult to remove. She should be advised that there is an increased risk of spontaneous abortion, premature labour or stillbirth. The IUD should be located after the birth if there are no complications.

If your client is not pregnant, then the threads may be found using either Spencer Wells forceps or a thread retriever like the Retrievette or the Emmett (Bounds et al., 1992b). If the threads are still lost, then an ultrasound should be performed to locate the position of the IUD. If the IUD is found to be correctly positioned in the uterus, then no further action is required. However, if it is not seen then a straight abdominal X-ray should be performed to exclude perforation.

- **PERFORATION:**

    If an IUD perforates the uterus, then it may also perforate the bowel or bladder, and an ultrasound and X-ray will need to be performed to locate the device and laparoscopy performed to remove the device.

    Perforation is rare and more common in post-partum lactating women who have IUDs fitted. It is important to encourage women to return if they have any pain or discomfort which persists following insertion.

- **INFECTION:**

    If a woman complains of any change in her normal discharge, such as vaginal itching, soreness, offensive and/or increased discharge or pain, then this should be investigated fully. If screening for all genital infections is unavailable, then you should refer women to their local genitourinary medicine clinic where screening for chlamydia and sexually transmitted diseases will be performed.

    Clients may wish to reduce the risk of infection by using condoms. Women may choose to use an IUD as a method of contraception and a condom to protect them against infection.

- **ECTOPIC PREGNANCY:**

    If a woman complains of low abdominal pain which may be associated with a light, scanty or missed period, then an ectopic pregnancy should be excluded. A pregnancy test and ultrasound will need to be performed to confirm the diagnosis; if this is confirmed, then she will need to be referred to her local hospital for emergency treatment.

- **PREGNANCY:**

    If a woman is pregnant with an intrauterine pregnancy and has an IUD in situ, then if she wishes to continue with the pregnancy, the IUD should be removed if the pregnancy is less than 12 weeks' gestation, the threads are visible and removal offers no resistance. There is a risk of spontaneous abortion if the IUD is removed but this is greater if the IUD is left in situ. *It is not always possible to remove the IUD. Removal should be attempted only by an experienced doctor following discussion with the client.*

- **PAIN OR BLEEDING:**

    If a woman complains of pain or bleeding with an IUD, then this should be investigated fully first to exclude infection, perforation or ectopic pregnancy. Details about the bleeding pattern or pain should be ascertained and a pregnancy test performed, along with a bimanual examination and cervical smear test, screening for infection and ultrasound scan. If the pain continues and infection, perforation and ectopic pregnancy have been excluded, then appropriate analgesia may be given, or the IUD may be changed. Changing an existing IUD to a different type of IUD may be a possible solution.

- **ACTINOMYCES-LIKE ORGANISMS:**

    Actinomyces-like organisms (ALOs) are bacteria found in women with IUDs in situ by cytologists when cervical screening is performed. If a woman is symptomatic, e.g. she complains of pain, dyspareunia or an increase in vaginal discharge, then sexually transmitted infections should be excluded, if on consultation with the woman the IUD is removed, this should be sent for culture, with the IUD threads removed, and a new IUD may be fitted. If the culture is negative to actinomyces, then a follow-up smear should be repeated. However, if the culture is positive to actinomyces, then she will require antibiotic therapy, which should be advised by the microbiology department (FSRH, 2023a).

> If your client is asymptomatic, the presence of ALOs does not necessitate removal of the device; however, careful counselling and follow-up should be discussed. After full counselling, your client will be able to make an informed decision about whether she wishes to have the IUD removed or left in situ. This decision should be documented in her notes.

SEXUALITY AND ANXIETIES

Women who choose the IUD as their form of contraception do so often because it is "out of sight and out of mind," meaning it requires little compliance or motivation from the woman and once in situ "can be forgotten." With an IUD, there is no disruption to sexual intercourse and, therefore, no loss of spontaneity. However, there are still many misconceptions held about IUDs by both men and women. Many people believe that the IUD causes infertility, infection and is an abortifacient. With such strong inaccurate views held, it is not surprising that many women do not consider it as an initial form of contraception; this highlights the need for comprehensive counselling.

Many women are unaware of new IUDs with higher efficacy and longer lifespans, which may take some women over difficult periods where other contraception is contraindicated and menopause is not too far off! Women may be concerned about the pain of insertion of an IUD. The use of pre-insertion analgesia and local anaesthetic can help to reduce this; however, the comfort and support of a nurse or a partner are vital.

A large proportion of women who have completed their families and do not wish to have any more choose to have an IUD fitted.

THE LEVONORGESTREL INTRAUTERINE DEVICE

Introduction

The levonorgestrel IUD (LNG-IUD) is licensed for contraception and for the treatment of primary menorrhagia, which has relieved many women from horrendous menstrual problems when the only previous solution would have been a hysterectomy.

Explanation of the method

The LNG-IUD has a plastic T-shaped frame with a steroid reservoir around the vertical stem of the device containing the progestogen hormone levonorgestrel. Mirena and Levosert contain 52 mg of levonorgestrel, whilst Kyleena contains 19.5 mg and Jaydess contains 13.5 mg. Mirena is impregnated with barium sulphate, which makes it radiopaque, and is licensed for five years (see Figure 8.2). Levosert is licensed for eight years. Kyleena is licensed for five years, and Jaydess which is a smaller LNG-IUD with a diameter of 3.8 mm and releases 13.5 mg of levonorgestrel over 24 hours, is licensed for three years.

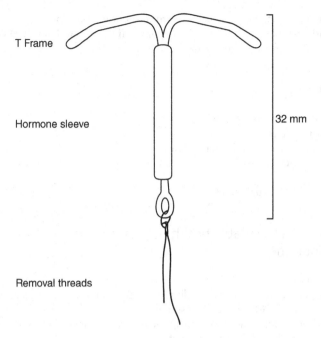

T Frame

Hormone sleeve

32 mm

Removal threads

Figure 8.2 LNG-IUD Mirena.

The LNG-IUD prevents pregnancy by the suppression of the endometrium, making it unfavourable to implantation. In some women, the LNG-IUD reduces ovarian function. It also causes the cervical mucus to thicken, making it impenetrable to sperm, and there is a foreign body reaction to the presence of the LNG-IUD.

Efficacy

The LNG- IUD, which contains 52 mg (Mirena and Levosert), has a failure rate of 99.8% in the first year of use (FRSH, 2023). The efficacy is 99.7% for the 19.5 mg and 13.5 mg LNG-IUD devices (Kyleena and Jaydess; FSRH, 2023). Whilst evidence shows that the LNG-IUD may be effective when it exceeds its license, using it beyond its license is not endorsed by the FSRH Clinical Effectiveness Unit (FSRH, 2023a).

Disadvantages

- Amenorrhoea
- Irregular bleeding
- Body of the LNG-IUD device is wider than other IUDs, which means that dilatation of cervix may be required
- Expulsion of the LNG-IUD
- Perforation of the uterus, bowel and bladder
- Malposition of the LNG-IUD

- Pregnancy caused by expulsion, perforation or malposition
- Slightly increased risk of ectopic pregnancy if there is an LNG-IUD failure
- Not suitable for post-coital use

Advantages

- Reduction in menorrhagia
- Reduction in dysmenorrhoea
- Oligomenorrhoea and amenorrhoea
- High efficacy
- Reversible
- Unrelated to sexual intercourse

UKMEC 4 unacceptable health risk – absolute contraindications

- Pregnancy
- Undiagnosed genital tract bleeding (once the cause has been diagnosed and treated, an LNG-IUD may be inserted)
- Pelvic or vaginal infection (symptomatic chlamydia or gonorrhoea; once treated, an LNG-IUD may be fitted)
- Post-partum sepsis
- Post-abortion sepsis
- Known pelvic tuberculosis
- Suspected or confirmed endometrial or cervical malignancy
- Current breast cancer
- Gestational trophoblastic disease with persistent elevated beta HCG levels or malignant disease
- Endometrial cancer
- Serious side effects occurring on the COC which are not due to oestrogen

UKMEC 3 risks outweigh the benefits of using method – relative contraindications

- Present liver disease, liver adenoma or cancer
- Current ischaemic heart disease, including TIA's and CVA
- Drugs which may interfere with the efficacy of the LNG-IUD, e.g. enzyme-inducing drugs
- Less than four weeks post-partum
- Congenital or acquired uterine anomaly which distorts the fundal cavity, like fibroids
- Past breast cancer in the last five years
- Organ transplant (for initiation)
- Known long QT syndrome (for initiation)
- HIV is classified as UKMEC3 for insertion if CD4 count < 200 and UKMEC2 for continuation; this is because of reduced immune system caused by the HIV virus and, as a result, an increased risk of infection

Range of method

At present, there are four types of LNG-IUD: Jaydess, Kyleena, Levosert and Mirena. Mirena and Levosert are the only LNG- IUDs licenced for eight years for contraception (FSRH, 2024a). Kyleena 19.5 mg LNG-IUD is licensed for five years and Jaydess 13.5 mg LNG-IUD for three years.

Mirena is the only devise licensed for five years for use in the prevention of endometrial hyperplasia and with oestrogen hormone placement therapy, and the treatment of menorrhagia. Levosert is licensed for five years for the treatment of menorrhagia (FSRH, 2023a).

Decision of choice

Women who are interested in having an LNG- IUD fitted should be carefully counselled about the side effects of the LNG-IUD. Functional ovarian cysts have been noted to be between 10% and 12% with the LNG-IUD (Robinson et al., 1989); most were asymptomatic and resolved spontaneously. The most common side effect the LNG-IUD is irregular bleeding patterns, whilst other side effects were found initially in the first few months following insertion. Research (Andersson et al., 1994; Sivin & Stern, 1994) has shown that the LNG-IUD significantly reduces bleeding and spotting and is particularly useful for women requiring contraception and treatment for menorrhagia and dysmenorrhoea (Bounds et al., 1993). Observational research has shown that Mirena has given significant symptomatic relief in women with adenomyosis (Ikoni, 2002).

When the LNG-IUD is removed, fertility returns to normal immediately and menstruation occurs within 30 days (Hollingworth & Guillebaud, 1994).

Side effects

- Some women may develop functional ovarian cysts
- Breast tenderness
- Acne
- Headaches
- Bloatedness
- Mood changes
- Nausea
- Irregular bleeding
- Amenorrhoea

Drugs which affect the efficacy of the LNG-IUD

The LNG-IUD releases progestogen directly into the uterus and is unaffected by metabolism of the liver, as a result, diarrhoea and vomiting, as well as drugs that alter gastric pH, will not reduce its effectiveness.

The LNG-IUD efficacy may be affected by progestogen receptor modulators such as ulipristal acetate and should not be quick started until five days afterwards and will not be effective for seven days after insertion (FSRH, 2023a).

The LNG-IUD efficacy is not reduced by griseofulvin, lamotrigine and enzyme-inducing drugs (FSRH, 2022, 2023a). However, as new enzyme drugs are developed, this should be checked for potential drug interaction via online drug interaction checker available on Stockley's Interaction Checker website, the British National Formulary online or via app or via the online HIV drugs interaction checker for Antiretroviral Therapy (ARV) drugs (https://www.hiv-druginteractions.org/checker). LNG-IUD effectiveness is not reduced by weight or BMI (FSRH, 2023a).

LNG-IUD counselling

As with any method of contraception, the more information given to a client will not only ensure that he or she chooses the best method but also increases their future acceptability of the method. When counselling your clients about the LNG-IUD, it is important to obtain a full medical history to exclude any contra-indications. The side effects and efficacy of the LNG-IUD should be discussed, along with your client's contraceptive history. It is important that up until inser-tion a reliable form of contraception is used, as the LNG-IUD is not licensed as emergency contraception.

Many women will choose to have the LNG-IUD inserted because of its high efficacy and therapeutic effects on menorrhagia and dysmenorrhoea, even if it may make their already present acne or breast tenderness worse. This is often because they feel that their contraception and periods are the greatest of these problems, and that they will, if necessary, put up with other problems to alleviate these. However, a woman who has very severe premenstrual problems and no problems with dysmenorrhoea or menorrhagia may find a Cu-IUD more suitable, as this will not increase her premenstrual symptoms.

To increase the acceptability and continuation rates with the LNG-IUD, it is important to discuss the hormonal side effects, such as mastalgia, headaches, acne, hirsutism and mood swings. Clients may choose to accept these side effects because of the advantages of the LNG-IUD; however, they should also be reminded that the amount of levonorgestrel received through the LNG-IUD is only a fraction of the daily dose received through oral contraceptives, so the side effects should be smaller with the LNG-IUD than with oral methods.

The LNG-IUD may cause oligomenorrhoea or amenorrhoea. There is a total reduction in menstrual blood loss because of the reduction in the thickness and vascularity of the endometrium caused by the presence of the LNG-IUD. This means that women may experience shorter, lighter, irregular menstrual periods and spotting. Spotting decreases with use and has been found to be less than four days at six months of use (Leiras, 1995). Women should be warned that they may experience amenorrhoea, which may cause some women anxiety; others, how-ever, may see this as an advantage.

The risks of LNG-IUD insertion procedure should be discussed, along with the choice of having local anaesthetic. It is important to talk about the possible need to dilate the cervix to introduce the LNG-IUD device, as this may be more painful than having an IUD inserted, and occasionally, the cervix will not dilate enough to allow insertion of the LNG-IUD, resulting in failure to fit the device. With all IUD and LNG-IUD procedures, there is a small risk of perforation of the uterus or cervix, 1–2 per 1000 insertions (FSRH, 2023a); however, with an experienced inserter, this risk will be lessened. There is a risk of partial or complete expulsion of the LNG-IUD, which is why it is important for it to have fundal positioning to reduce this possibility.

It is important to counsel your client about the possible risks if she becomes pregnant with an intrauterine pregnancy with the LNG-IUD in situ. Because of the high efficacy of the device, there is limited information available about the outcome of a pregnancy with the LNG-IUD. Because of the local exposure to levonorgestrel of an intrauterine pregnancy, teratogenicity and virilisation cannot be excluded, and termination of the pregnancy should be discussed. If this is discussed at counselling, then women can think about this issue, and if they hold strong views against abortion, they may wish to choose another method.

Prior to insertion of the LNG-IUD, a bimanual examination should be performed to exclude any abnormalities of the uterine cavity such as fibroids, which will necessitate an ultrasound scan to confirm diagnosis prior to insertion. If a fibroid is causing the uterine cavity to be distorted, then the LNG-IUD will be contraindicated. Screening for chlamydia and gonorrhoea should be performed at this examination. If there is any suspicion of a genitourinary infection, a full screening should be performed; if this is unavailable, then your client will need to be referred to a genitourinary clinic. The use of prophylactic antibiotics with immunocompromised women should be assessed individually and discussed with their consultants (FSRH, 2023a).

The areas to be covered at counselling are summarized in Box 8.2.

Box 8.2

Areas to be covered during counselling

- Full medical history
- Check blood pressure, weight and height
- Ensure client has contraceptive cover up to insertion
- Take details of last menstrual period; exclude pregnancy
- Discuss how an LNG-IUD works and its efficacy
- Discuss insertion and removal procedure
- Discuss side effects, e.g. amenorrhoea, irregular menstrual cycle
- Discuss risks of insertion – expulsion, perforation, pregnancy and ectopic pregnancy
- Perform bimanual examination to exclude contraindications and take chlamydia and gonorrhoea swab
- Discuss safer sex
- Give literature on LNG-IUD

LNG-IUD insertion procedure

Prior to insertion of the LNG-IUD, chlamydia and gonorrhoea result should be checked, information about the last menstrual period should be obtained to exclude an already present pregnancy and a pregnancy test performed if required, as the LNG-IUD is not licensed as an emergency contraceptive. It is therefore important to exclude any unprotected sexual intercourse, as the LNG-IUD cannot be fitted if there is any risk of pregnancy. Fitting of the LNG-IUD is like that of the IUD. Research (Guillebaud and Bounds 1983) has shown that if mefenamic acid 500 mg is given orally prior to insertion, there is a reduction in pain following insertion of an IUD. Women should empty their bladders prior to insertion, as this will make it easier for the inserter to feel the uterus abdominally, and it will be more comfortable for the woman. Emergency equipment should be available at all LNG-IUD and IUD insertion procedures (see p. 120–121).

During the LNG-IUD insertion procedure, your client may like to have someone to comfort her. Prior to insertion, a bimanual examination will be performed by the inserter to ascertain the size, position, and direction of the uterus, and to check that there is no tenderness.

Your client may like to have local anaesthetic to reduce pain, as the cervix may need to be dilated to fit the LNG-IUD. Anaesthesia can be given with a paracervical block using lignocaine.

As an LNG-IUD insertion may involve dilatation of the cervix to introduce the device, the procedure should be carried out by an inserter who has received further training in LNG-IUD insertion and paracervical anaesthesia.

Insertion of an LNG-IUD is performed by a "non-touch technique," so a clean pair of gloves should be used following bimanual examination. A sterile speculum is inserted into the vagina, and the cervix is located; this is then cleaned with sterile cotton wool and antiseptic solution. A uterine sound is inserted into the uterus via the cervical canal to measure the length, direction and patency of the uterus. This may cause cramp-like period pains, which should diminish when the uterine sound is removed. The cervix may be stabilised by Allis forceps or a tenaculum so that the LNG-IUD may be inserted more easily; these may cause some discomfort, as the cervix is very sensitive. As the introducer to the LNG-IUD is wider than other IUDs, Hegar dilators may need to be used to dilate the cervix to Hegar 5 or 6 in diameter. This may be uncomfortable, and local anaesthetic can help to alleviate this discomfort. Next, the LNG-IUD is inserted through the cervical canal into the uterus. The threads of the LNG-IUD are shortened once it is in position and are tucked up behind the cervix. Fundal positioning of the LNG-IUD is extremely important to reduce the risk of expulsion and to ensure the endometrium has full exposure to the progestogen in the device and maximum efficacy is obtained.

Following insertion of the LNG-IUD, you should encourage your client to lie down and rest. Analgesia may be required for period pains. Sanitary towels should be used initially to reduce the risk of infection and because tampons may catch on the LNG-IUD threads which have not yet softened. Tampons may be used with the next menstrual period. Your client may experience bleeding initially; this is a good time to remind her of any initial problems and when to return — for example, if she experiences a change in her normal vaginal discharge or persistent abdominal pain.

You should teach your client how to check her LNG-IUD threads and encourage her to perform this after each menstrual period. It is helpful to show your client a picture of the LNG-IUD and give up-to-date written information, along with relevant telephone numbers of where to get help if needed. It is recommended that the LNG-IUD is fitted within the first five days of the onset of menstruation with no additional contraception required, if fitted at any other time additional contraception is required for seven days (FSRH, 2023a). An LNG-IUD procedure usually takes ten minutes. The batch number of the LNG-IUD device and expiry date should be recorded in the woman's notes. Ideally, you will see your client in four to six weeks for an initial follow-up after insertion. Your client should be advised to return earlier if she experiences pain, unusual vaginal discharge or pyrexia.

The LNG-IUD can be inserted immediately following a first trimester abortion and should be inserted within 48 hours after childbirth or from 4 weeks after childbirth if pregnancy has been excluded (FSRH, 2023a).

LNG-IUD removal procedure

Removal of the LNG-IUD is the same as removing an IUD; clients should not have had sexual intercourse within the last seven days. As fertility returns immediately, contraception should be discussed prior to removal, e.g. diaphragm should be taught and fitted or oral contraception commenced prior to removal if wanted.

Subsequent visits

Following insertion of the LNG-IUD, an examination should be performed four to six weeks later, when blood pressure and weight should be taken. Details about menstrual cycle and any problems experienced should be ascertained. If your client has had amenorrhoea since fitting, then a pregnancy test should be performed to exclude pregnancy; however, if there are no symptoms and the device is in situ, then you can reassure your client. A speculum and bimanual examination should be performed to check that the device is correctly positioned. The LNG-IUD threads should be visible on speculum examination. If the end of the LNG-IUD device is felt (it feels like the end of a matchstick), then the device is partially expelled. This is a good opportunity to show your client how to check her threads for the LNG-IUD if she is unable to do so.

If there are no problems and the device is correctly positioned, you should remind your client when to return early – for example, if she experiences any persistent abdominal pain, unusual discharge, pyrexia or symptoms of pregnancy, or if she is in any way concerned.

PROBLEMS ENCOUNTERED

■ LOST THREADS:

If you or your client are unable to feel the LNG-IUD threads this may indicate that the LNG-IUD has been expelled or that it has moved within the uterus or perforated the uterus taking the threads with it. You should advise your client to use alternative contraception, as she may be at risk of pregnancy. However, she may already be pregnant, and a pregnancy test should be performed to exclude this, along with details of her last menstrual period and any signs of pregnancy which may be experienced. Extrauterine pregnancy should be excluded first by an ultrasound scan. If your client has an intrauterine pregnancy, then careful counselling will need to be given.

If your client is not pregnant, then the threads may be found using either Spencer Wells forceps or a thread retriever. If the threads are still lost, then an ultrasound should be performed to locate the position of the LNG-IUD. If the LNG-IUD is found to be correctly positioned in the uterus, then no further action is required. However, if it is not seen, then a straight abdominal X-ray should be performed to exclude perforation.

■ PERFORATION:

If an LNG-IUD perforates the uterus, then it may also perforate the bowel or bladder, and an ultrasound, and X-rays will need to be performed to locate the device and laparoscopy performed to remove the device. It is important to encourage women to return if they have any pain or discomfort which persists following insertion.

■ ECTOPIC PREGNANCY:

If a woman complains of low abdominal pain which may be associated with a light, scanty or missed period, then an ectopic pregnancy should be excluded. A pregnancy test and ultrasound will need to be performed to confirm diagnosis. If this is confirmed, then she will need to be referred to her local hospital for emergency treatment.

■ PREGNANCY:

If a woman is pregnant with an intrauterine pregnancy and has an LNG-IUD in situ, then careful counselling will need to be given about the possible risk of teratogenicity and virilisation in the foetus, due to local exposure to levonorgestrel. Due to a lack of clinical experience with pregnancies with an LNG-IUD in situ, information is limited, and a termination of pregnancy should be discussed with your client.

■ PAIN:

If a woman complains of pain or bleeding with an LNG-IUD, then this should be investigated fully to exclude infection, perforation or ectopic pregnancy. Details about the bleeding pattern and pain should be ascertained, and a pregnancy test performed along with a bimanual examination and cervical smear test, screening for infection and an ultrasound scan.

■ ACTINOMYCES-LIKE ORGANISMS (ALOs):

ALOs are bacteria found in women with LNG-IUD in situ by cytologists when cervical screening is performed. If a woman is symptomatic, e.g. she complains of pain, dyspareunia or an increase in vaginal discharge, then the LNG-IUD may be removed and sent for culture and STI screen completed, and a new LNG-IUD fitted. If the culture is negative to actinomyces, then a follow-up smear should be repeated. However, if the culture is positive to actinomyces, then she will require antibiotic therapy, which should be advised by the microbiology department (FSRH, 2023a).

However, if your client is asymptomatic, the presence of ALOs does not necessitate removal of the device. Careful counselling ensuring that there are no symptoms which do necessitate removal and follow-up should be discussed. After full counselling, your client will be able to make an informed decision about whether she wishes to have the LNG-IUD removed or left in situ. This decision should be documented in her notes.

■ HEAVIER OR INCREASED MENSTRUAL BLEEDING:

Heavier or increased menstrual bleeding may indicate a partial expulsion of the LNG-IUD, as the endometrium may not have full exposure to levonorgestrel; there will also be a decrease in efficacy of the device. You should advise your client to use alternative contraception, e.g. condom. She should have a bimanual and speculum examination and a pregnancy test to exclude partial or complete expulsion and pregnancy. If this is not excluded, then an ultrasound should be performed to locate the device.

SELF-ASSESSMENT QUESTIONS

Answers and discussion at the end of the chapter.

4 A 24-year-old woman consults requesting contraception after being refused a sterilisation because of her age. She has three children and has had two miscarriages. None of her pregnancies have been planned, and she finds it difficult to remember to take pills. What forms of contraception would be suitable for her?
5 What are the advantages of the LNG-IUD to a woman?
6 Who would be most suitable for LNG-IUD, and who do you think would be less suitable for an LNG-IUD and why?

SEXUALITY AND ANXIETIES

With the introduction of the LNG-IUD, the field of contraception has widened considerably. Not only does the LNG-IUD offer an extremely effective form of contraception, but it also offers many women treatment for dysmenorrhoea and menorrhagia; for many of these women, the only relief of these symptoms would have been to have a hysterectomy. LNG-IUD also offers women a suitable reversible option to sterilisation and has given women who are unable to use combined oral contraception another acceptable choice.

Many women who consult requesting LNG-IUD have complex gynaecological and sexual histories – they perceive the LNG-IUD as being the answer to all their problems, which it may well be! Often, these women have tried all methods of contraception in an effort to solve their problems, with no success. However, some of these problems may be of a psychosexual nature, which the LNG-IUD will not alleviate. Given time these anxieties may surface; if, however they are not expressed, they may appear as feelings of dissatisfaction with the method.

ANSWERS TO SELF-ASSESSMENT QUESTIONS

1 Your client, who has an IUD in situ, is concerned that her menstrual period is two weeks late. What would you do?

It is important to exclude pregnancy when your client has a delayed menstrual period. Details of the last episode of sexual intercourse and last menstrual period should be ascertained, and a pregnancy test performed if required. If your client is at risk of pregnancy and the test is negative, then she will need to have a bimanual examination and ultrasound scan to exclude extrauterine or intrauterine pregnancy. If these are all negative, then your client may be reassured that she is not pregnant. If the test is positive, then she will need to have an ultrasound scan to exclude extrauterine pregnancy. If the pregnancy is an ectopic pregnancy, then your client will need to be referred to the local hospital for emergency surgery. Once an extrauterine pregnancy has been excluded depending on how your client feels about the pregnancy, then this will determine her care. If she does not wish to proceed with the pregnancy and wishes to have a termination of pregnancy, then the IUD may be removed at the time of the termination procedure. If your client wishes to continue with the pregnancy and is under 12 weeks gestation, then the IUD may be removed following discussion of the risks with her if removal offers no resistance.

2 A 45-year-old woman attends for her IUD to be changed. It was inserted five years ago and is a Novaplus T 380. What would you do in this situation, and what further information do you need to know?

On discussion with the woman, it may be decided to leave the IUD in situ longer. Information about keeping devices in past their licence should be given so that she can make an informed decision.

It may be useful to find out when the woman's mother went through the menopause as this may give an indication as to when she may do so. This will give a very rough idea on how long she will require contraception for. It is also important to find out how she feels about pregnancy and whether it will cause her more anxiety by not changing the IUD.

3 A 35-year-old woman consults complaining of dyspareunia for two months. She is in a permanent relationship and has had an IUD in situ for two years with no previous problems. What would you do in this situation?

It is important to find out more about the dyspareunia. Has there been a change in the women's discharge? Does she have pain at any other time? How long has she had dyspareunia? Can she describe the pain when she gets it?

She will need to be examined to exclude infection and to check the IUD. A bimanual and screening for all infections should be performed. If these are unavailable, then she will need to be referred. Until infection has been excluded, she should be advised to use condoms to protect her partner against infection.

Once infection has been excluded and the IUD has been checked to be in the correct position, then other causes of dyspareunia need to be investigated. There may be a psychosexual aspect to the dyspareunia which may need to be explored. Has the woman's relationship changed? Has she had dyspareunia before? Given time, this client may be able to talk about this difficult area.

4   A 24-year-old woman consults requesting contraception after being refused a sterilisation because of her age. She has three children and has had two miscarriages. None of her pregnancies have been planned and she finds it difficult to remember to take pills. What forms of contraception would be suitable for her?

From this history, the client is looking for a method of contraception which has a high efficacy and which does not require compliance, as she finds it difficult to remember to take oral contraception. There are several methods available to her which fit this description – Depo-Provera, IUDs and the LNG-IUD. Careful counselling should be given about each method and a detailed medical history taken so that an informed decision may be made by the client. Some women may choose not to have Depo-Provera because of the requirement of having injections every 11–12 weeks. An IUD which has an eight-year licence or an LNG-IUD may be a good choice; both offer high efficacy and little client compliance.

5   What are the advantages of the LNG-IUD to a woman?

The main advantages of the LNG-IUD to a woman are that her periods will become less painful and lighter; she may also experience no periods. If a woman has experienced anaemia from heavy periods, this will also be alleviated. The LNG-IUD offers highly effective contraception with very low pregnancy rates, with the added benefit of being completely reversible. Lastly, the LNG-IUD requires little compliance from a woman and is unrelated to sexual intercourse.

6   Who would be most suitable for an LNG-IUD, and who do you think would be less suitable for an LNG-IUD and why?

Those most suitable for the LNG-IUD are the following types of women:

■   Those requesting a method of contraception for a five-year period or more.
■   Women who want a method with a high efficacy; they may have had a contraceptive failure or do not wish to become pregnant.
■   Those who may suffer from heavy or painful periods.
■   Women who may be unable to use other methods of contraception because of contraindications, e.g. they have focal migraines and are unable to have the COC, or they may be unable to have the IUD due to heavy periods.
■   Women who are less suitable for the LNG-IUD include those who have experienced side effects with progestogen methods. These women may find the menstrual disturbances unacceptable. Some women find it disturbing to have amenorrhoea, as this usually is an indicator of pregnancy. Women are unable to have the LNG-IUD fitted if they are pregnant, have undiagnosed genital tract bleeding or have a suspected malignancy or liver disorder. Women who have an abnormality of the uterus which distorts the uterus may be unable to have the LNG-IUD because the device may be expelled more easily. Women with circulatory disorders, thromboembolic disease, heart valve replacement and history of bacterial endocarditis should be reviewed individually, and specialist consultant advice sought. Other contraindications are women who have had recent trophoblastic disease, ischaemic heart disease or who are taking drugs which may interfere with the efficacy of the LNG-IUD.

9

EMERGENCY CONTRACEPTION

INTRODUCTION

There are three types of emergency contraception: two hormonal and one non-hormonal. The two hormonal emergency contraceptives licensed in the UK are the levonorgestrel emergency contraception (LNG-EC) method, which is available in the form of Levonelle One or Levonelle 1500, and the ulipristal acetate emergency contraception (UPA-EC) method, which is provided in the form of ellaOne. Levonelle One and ellaOne are available over the counter in chemists. A Copper intrauterine device (Cu- IUD) may be inserted as a post-coital method, but this is not generally as well-known as an emergency hormonal method among the general public or professionals.

Prior to giving emergency contraception, it is important to take a full medical history, including medications and allergies. In order to ascertain what method the client is eligible for, you will need to have detailed information about the date of the last menstrual period, and when the client has had unprotected sexual intercourse and earlier emergency contraception administered this cycle.

Emergency contraception has two main methods: hormonal contraception and intrauterine contraception. The copper intrauterine device (Cu-IUD) is the most effective method in preventing pregnancy followed by the UPA-EC method, and finally the LNG-EC method.

INTRAUTERINE CONTRACEPTIVE DEVICES

Explanation of the method

A Cu-IUD works as a post-coital method by preventing implantation and may also block fertilisation. A Cu-IUD can be inserted up to five days after the first unprotected sexual intercourse (UPSI) in a natural menstrual cycle or up to five days after the earliest likely calculated date of ovulation, whichever is later (FSRH, March 2017a, amended July 2023). As pregnancy and implantation do not occur until five to seven days after fertilisation, this means that the Cu-IUD does not act as an abortifacient.

Efficacy

The Cu-IUD is almost 100% effective in preventing pregnancy post coitally.

DOI: 10.4324/9781003484424-10

Disadvantages

- Slightly increased risk of ectopic pregnancy if there is a Cu-IUD failure
- Increased risk of pelvic infection
- Expulsion of the Cu-IUD
- Perforation of the uterus, bowel and bladder (this risk is raised in breast feeding women; FSRH, March 2017a, amended July 2023)
- Malposition of the Cu-IUD
- Pregnancy caused by expulsion, perforation or malposition
- Minor surgical procedure

Advantages

- Effective in preventing pregnancy
- Unrelated to partner
- Cu-IUD may be kept *in situ* and used as a form of contraception for the future
- Longer time span of up to five days

UKMEC 4 unacceptable health risk – absolute contraindications

- Pregnancy
- Present pelvic, vaginal infection, although a Cu-IUD may be inserted in special circumstances with antibiotic cover
- Undiagnosed genital tract bleeding
- Persistently elevated beta human chorionic gonadotrophin (HCG) levels or malignant disease; a Cu-IUD should not be inserted
- Less than four weeks post-partum a Cu-IUD should not be inserted

Range of method

A Cu-IUD is used for post-coital emergency contraception.

Side effects

- Menorrhagia
- Dysmenorrhoea
- A Cu-IUD may be difficult to fit in nulliparous women

Decision of choice

A Cu-IUD may be fitted as a form of emergency contraception up to five days after the calculated date of ovulation. It provides contraception for the rest of the month, and if a woman wishes can either be left *in situ* after her next menstrual period or be removed. Women who have a contraindication to the hormonal method may be able to have a Cu-IUD fitted, along with women who cannot accept the failure rate of the hormonal method.

Counselling

Women who have a post-coital Cu-IUD fitted may be more anxious than women having a routine Cu-IUDs fitted, which can make insertion difficult. As they have had less time to prepare themselves for the procedure, it is important to allow them time to ask any questions and discuss the insertion procedure, risks, efficacy and advantages and disadvantages of the Cu-IUD. You should complete a full medical history which will enable you to eliminate and contraindications to the procedure and, with the aid of a menstrual calendar and information on the first day of the last menstrual period, estimate the calculated date of ovulation. If there is any possibility of your client being pregnant, you should complete a pregnancy test, and a bimanual examination will need to be performed to exclude pregnancy.

If your client has not eaten recently, it is preferable that she has something to eat prior to insertion; this will reduce the chances of her feeling faint. Analgesia may be given and will be absorbed faster if a client has eaten. Although all this may seem time-consuming, it will have the effect of reducing anxiety in the woman which will aid insertion of the device and will reduce pain felt following insertion.

Prior to fitting a Cu-IUD, ideally, screening for chlamydia and gonorrhoea should be performed. As the result will not be available for the insertion of a post-coital Cu-IUD, prophylactic antibiotics are not recommended. If there are signs of cervical or pelvic infection, full screening for infection is recommended, especially in the case of rape, which may necessitate referral to a genitourinary medicine (GUM) clinic. When referring your client to a GUM clinic, you may find it possible for the post-coital Cu-IUD to be inserted following screening at the clinic.

The Cu-IUD procedure is the same as for a routine Cu-IUD procedure. The client should be shown how to check her Cu-IUD threads and be advised that she may experience some bleeding and period-like pains after fitting. She should be encouraged to avoid tampons and use sanitary towels immediately after insertion in case these catch on the threads. If she experiences persistent pain, she should be advised to seek medical attention to exclude an ectopic pregnancy. It is vital to give up-to-date literature and emergency telephone numbers to your client. A follow-up appointment should be made three to four weeks following insertion.

Follow-up appointment

You should see your client three to four weeks following insertion to check that she has had a normal menstrual period. If this is shorter or lighter than normal, a pregnancy test should be performed to exclude pregnancy. If she is having her Cu-IUD removed with her period, then alternative contraception should be commenced seven days prior to removal. Hormonal contraception is usually commenced on day 1 of a normal period. The COC should be commenced on day 1 of a normal menstrual period with no additional precautions required. The POP should be commenced on day 1 of a normal menstrual period with no additional precautions required. Once alternative contraception has been established, then the Cu-IUD may be removed. If, however, she would like to continue with the Cu-IUD as her method of contraception, the Cu-IUD should be checked.

HORMONAL EMERGENCY CONTRACEPTION

There are two types of hormonal contraception:

- Ulipristal acetate method (UPA-EC).
- Levonorgestrel method (LNG-EC).

ULIPRISTAL ACETATE METHOD (UPA-EC).

Explanation of the method

Ulipristal acetate prevents pregnancy by inhibiting or delaying ovulation depending on when in the cycle it is administered. It is believed that ulipristal acetate can prevent ovulation after the luteal surge has started and delay follicular rupture up to five days later. If ulipristal acetate is administered after implantation has occurred, there is limited evidence on the effects on pregnancy and teratogenicity.

Ulipristal acetate is a synthetic progesterone which binds to human progesterone receptor; as a result, it blocks the action of progestogen and may reduce the efficacy of contraceptives containing progestogen. Ulipristal acetate has a high affinity for glucocorticoid receptor, and anti-glucocorticoid effects have been observed in animals. It is therefore not recommended for use with women suffering from severe asthma insufficiently controlled by oral glucocorticoids (FSRH, March 2017a, amended July 2023).

Efficacy

Ulipristal acetate is the most effective emergency hormonal method within the first 120 hours after UPSI and is between 99% and 98% effective (FSRH, March 2017a, amended July 2023). However, all hormonal methods are ineffective if taken after ovulation (FSRH, March 2017a, amended July 2023).

Disadvantages

- Does not provide future contraception
- Next menstrual period may be early or delayed
- Nausea and vomiting

Advantages

- Effective in preventing pregnancy
- Under the woman's control

UKMEC 4 unacceptable health risk – absolute contraindications

- Pregnancy
- Allergy to constituents
- Severe asthma controlled by glucocorticoids

- Repeated doses in the same cycle
- Galactose intolerance and Lapp lactose deficiency or glucose-galactose mal-absorption as UPA-EC contains lactose

Range of method

Ulipristal acetate method contains 30 mg of ulipristal acetate and is given within 120 hours of UPSI. It is licensed under the name ellaOne. It is available in the form of ellaOne for post-coital use, with an instruction leaflet over the counter from pharmacists for £30 and free from sexual health clinics, walk-in centres and general practitioners.

Side effects

- Nausea
- Vomiting
- Fatigue
- Headaches
- Menstrual disorders

HOW TO TAKE THE ULIPRISTAL ACETATE METHOD

The ulipristal acetate method is prescribed as ellaOne contains one tablet. One tablet should be taken within 120 hours from the earliest episode of UPSI. As emergency contraception can make women feel nauseated, it is a good idea to advise them to take the tablet with or after food.

If the client vomits within three hours after taking ellaOne, then she will need to return for a repeat prescription and take the dose immediately within the 120 hours. If a woman suffers from severe vomiting, then a Cu-IUD may need to be considered. The FSRH state that there is no longer any need to disrupt breast feeding following a single dose of ulipristal acetate FSRH 2025).

DRUGS WHICH AFFECT THE EFFICACY OF THE ULIPRISTAL ACETATE METHOD

Liver enzyme–inducing drugs may reduce the efficacy of hormonal emergency contraception. In this situation a Cu-IUD should be first choice of emergency contraception. If a Cu-IUD is not appropriate women should be warned that LNG-EC and UPA-EC have reduced effectiveness. However, the FSRH recommends that Levonelle 1.5 mg is increased by 100%, so a stat dose orally of Levonelle 3 mg two 1.5 mg tablets should be given within 72 hours (FSRH, March 2017a, amended July 2023). The current advice with liver enzyme–inducing drugs and ulipristal acetate is that it is not used whilst a woman is taking these drugs or within 28 days after they have been used. The Clinical Effectiveness Unit does not recommend increasing the dose of ulipristal acetate (FSRH, March 2017a, amended July 2023).

Ulipristal acetate's effectiveness is reduced in women who have taken progestogen prior to it. Progestogen-containing contraception should not be commenced until five days after taking ulipristal acetate, as this will reduce its effectiveness (FSRH, March 2017a, amended July 2023).

Ulipristal acetate has been shown to be affected by the use of esomeprazole, a proton pump inhibitor, but the clinical significance is unknown and there is no current advice (FSRH, March 2017a, amended July 2023).

THE LEVONORGESTREL METHOD

Explanation of the method

The levonorgestrel method prevents pregnancy if taken prior to the luteal surge by inhibiting or delaying ovulation. The levonorgestrel method has been shown to be less ineffective if taken after ovulation (FSRH, March 2017a, amended July 2023). There is no evidence of any pregnancy complications or congenital malformations associated with this method.

Efficacy

The efficacy of the levonorgestrel method has been found to be 97%–99% but has in some studies been found to be as low as 85% effective in preventing pregnancy (FSRH, March 2017a, amended July 2023). Both hormonal methods have been found to be ineffective if taken after ovulation (FSRH, March 2017a, amended July 2023).

Disadvantages

- Does not provide future contraception
- Next menstrual period may be early or delayed
- Nausea and vomiting

Advantages

- Effective in preventing pregnancy
- Under the woman's control

UKMEC 4 unacceptable health risk – absolute contraindications

- Pregnancy
- However, the UK Medical Eligibility Criteria advise that there are no medical contraindications to the levonorgestrel method but caution should be applied to women with acute active porphyria, severe liver disease and allergy to levonorgestrel (FSRH, March 2017a, amended July 2023)

Range of method

Levonelle 1500 has one tablet made of the hormone progestogen, containing 1.5 mg of levonorgestrel. It is available in the form of Levonelle One for post-coital use, with an instruction leaflet over the counter from pharmacists from £10 to £20 and free from sexual health clinics, walk-in centres and general practitioners.

The levonorgestrel method should be commenced within 72 hours of the earliest episode of UPSI.

Side effects

- Nausea
- Vomiting
- Fatigue
- Headaches
- Dizziness
- Breast tenderness

How to take the levonorgestrel method

The levonorgestrel method is prescribed as Levonelle One or Levonelle 1500. Schering Levonelle One and Levonelle 1500 contain one tablet. One tablet should be taken within 72 hours from the earliest episode of UPSI. As emergency contraception can make women feel nauseated, it is a good idea to advise them to take the tablet with or after food.

If the client vomits within 3 hours after taking Schering Levonelle One, then she will need to return for a repeat prescription and take the dose immediately within 72 hours. If a woman suffers from severe vomiting, then a Cu-IUD may need to be considered.

Drugs which affect the efficacy of the levonorgestrel method regimen

It is believed that enzyme-inducing drugs like rifampicin may reduce the effect of emergency hormonal contraception and LNG-EC; it is currently recommended that a Cu-IUD is offered as the most effective form of emergency contraception. Two tablets of Levonelle 1500 (1.5 mg of levonorgestrel) may be given, increasing the dose to one stat dose of 3 mg of Levonelle 1500, although this is outside the product licence, so it would need to be unlicensed prescribing and the effectiveness is unknown (FSRH, March 2017a, amended July 2023).

How do you decide between hormonal emergency contraception?

The hormonal emergency methods are safe and effective methods. Deciding which method to choose is made once a careful history has been taken and detailed counselling given. It is important to ascertain when UPSI has taken place. A Cu-IUD is the most effective method, followed by ulipristal acetate and the levonorgestrel method. If a woman has an absolute contraindication to the hormonal method, then a Cu-IUD should be considered. Women wishing to use the CU-IUD as a method of contraception may have this fitted as an emergency method; however, it is important to remember that occasionally a Cu-IUD is unable to be inserted, and if this is the case, it may be more likely to occur with nulliparous women. Another factor to remember when choosing which method to use is the risk of genitourinary infection, which may be the result of the UPSI. Because of this factor, if the episode is within 72 hours, then taking the hormonal method may be of less risk to the woman than fitting a Cu-IUD.

Ulipristal acetate is the next most effective method after a Cu-IUD but may not be suitable if a woman has recently taken progestogen or had emergency hormonal contraception. The FSRH state that there is no longer any need to disrupt breast feeding following a single dose of ulipristal acetate FSRH.2025). The levonorgestrel method may be given more than once in the cycle, whereas ulipristal acetate is not recommended. There may be occasions when a client is unsuitable for a post-coital Cu-IUD; for example, if a woman has PID or has been raped or feels unable to go through the procedure of an insertion and is unable to have ulipristal acetate, giving the levonorgestrel method late may then be indicated.

COUNSELLING

Women who attend for emergency contraception are often very anxious and embarrassed; they may show varying emotions from anger to guilt. Sexual intercourse may not have been with consent, and she may feel shocked and distressed. Often, the situations women find themselves in feel threatening to them, and their feelings of anger, guilt, etc., are aimed at you. You may come across women who have difficulty in answering some of the personal questions you need to ask. "Why do you need to know that?" is not an uncommon response. It is important to allow enough time for this consultation and explain why you need to ask such personal questions. It is also a good idea to allow your client time to read through up-to-date literature about emergency contraception beforehand so that you can build on this knowledge and answer any questions this may initiate.

Often, clients fail to tell you about earlier episodes of UPSI, as they do not feel they are at risk of pregnancy from these episodes. Women often believe that UPSI around the end of their menstrual period will be safe, so this can be a good opportunity to explain about ovulation and how it is possible for sperm to live in the body for up to five to seven days. It may be possible to fit a Cu-IUD if a woman has had multiple episodes of unprotected intercourse and they are within five days of calculated date of ovulation. It is useful when taking details about episodes of earlier UPSI to chart these on a menstrual calendar, along with details of when the first day of the last menstrual period occurred and length of normal menstrual cycle; this will also make calculating ovulation easier. Often, whilst you are doing this, it triggers clients' memories, and they remember further episodes of UPSI.

If there is any doubt that your client's last menstrual period was not normal, then a pregnancy test should be performed to exclude pregnancy. Some women mistakenly believe that emergency contraception will be effective in preventing an existing pregnancy.

When counselling men and women about emergency contraception, it is important to discuss the efficacy and side effects of post-coital contraception. Sometimes women decide not to have emergency contraception after they have received counselling; this usually happens when the woman is in a stable relationship and willing to accept the risk of pregnancy or if the risk is low. Occasionally, it is not possible to give post-coital contraception because the woman has had multiple episodes of UPSI which exceed 120 hours and are beyond 5 days of calculated ovulation, so a Cu-IUD is unable to be inserted. This situation is often made worse if the woman has had UPSI with someone other than her regular partner. As health professionals you want to make "everything better." This is a situation when you are unable to do this, and this can be very difficult not only for the client but also for the nurse. What you may find hardest is that you can give no guarantees: you cannot reassure the woman that she won't become pregnant because there is a real risk that she may become pregnant. You also need to approach the issue of safer sex and contraception, which may at this time be an area she has not thought of. Listening to the woman's distress and anxieties is a main function of the nurse. It is often hard not to falsely reassure a woman in this situation but being there and listening to the pain your client is suffering are far more important to her. An appointment should be made after your client's estimated next menstrual period so that a pregnancy test can be performed; if possible, this appointment should be with you.

Sometimes the request for emergency contraception has been precipitated by rape. Shock may stop a woman from attending early for emergency contraception, which may mean that a Cu-IUD is indicated or that you are unable to give emergency contraception. It is vital that a woman has screening for all genitourinary infections and HIV from a specialist clinic. Rape counselling should be offered. Women may feel that they do not want this at the time, but information and telephone numbers should be given in case they wish to follow this up in the future.

Many different women and men attend for emergency contraception. They may be women in their 40s whose UPSI may cause a change in their contraceptive practice to a permanent method like sterilisation in the future; they may feel that they should know better and be embarrassed. Other clients may be young men and women who may be under the age of 16 and recently commenced sexual activity. They may be anxious that the information they give may not stay confidential, embarrassed and humiliated by the personal questions that are asked. Many younger clients feel that they will be judged by the health professionals they see. It has usually taken a great deal of courage for them to attend, and the impression they gain from this encounter will establish whether they attend in the future. Their confidentiality should be respected unless the health, safety or welfare of someone other than the client is at serious risk (BMA et al., 1993). Occasionally, young clients are being sexually abused, and if given time for a rapport to establish, they may return to confide in you.

A full medical history of the client and family should be completed to exclude any contraindications. If a client has previously had emergency contraception, it is useful to know if she had any problems such as vomiting so that appropriate advice can be given. If a woman has used emergency contraception repeatedly because of a contraceptive failure or because no contraception has been used, then future contraception should be discussed carefully. If your client has had a contraceptive failure, teaching them how to avoid this in the future will help reduce the necessity of emergency contraception in the future.

It is extremely important that women continue to use either a condom or abstain until their next period, as hormonal emergency contraception will not stop a woman from becoming pregnant in the remaining part of the cycle. If a woman has a further episode of UPSI, then she may be more at risk of pregnancy, because emergency methods can delay ovulation, resulting in this episode now being when she is ovulating! Women should be advised that if this situation occurs, they need to return for further treatment. There is often a great deal of anxiety about giving repeated doses of hormonal emergency contraception, but as along as the latest episode is within 72 hours and there are no other contraindications, then the levonorgestrel method may be prescribed.

ACTIVITY

Do you know where your clients can receive emergency contraception if you are unavailable? What about weekends and bank holidays?

Blood pressure, height and weight should be checked; a pelvic examination is not required with the hormonal method unless pregnancy is suspected or screening for infection is suspected. Anyone who has UPSI puts themselves at risk of sexually transmitted disease and HIV, and if full infection screening is unavailable, then they should be referred to their local GUM clinic.

When giving emergency contraception to clients, it is important to explore their attitudes towards pregnancy and discuss the possible failure of emergency contraception. There is no evidence to indicate that levonorgestrel and ulipristal methods are teratogenic if taken in early pregnancy (FSRH, March 2017a, amended July 2023). However, no one can guarantee a normal outcome to any pregnancy.

You should advise your client that her next menstrual period may be early, on time or later than expected. If it is not a normal period or is absent, she should return with a urine sample so that a pregnancy test can be performed. There is a risk in early pregnancy of an ectopic pregnancy. If a woman experiences abdominal pain, she should be advised to seek medical attention. It is good practice to offer women the opportunity to return three to four weeks later; this gives you the opportunity to review any problems with contraception.

As clients are often very anxious when they consult, all the information you give should be backed up by up-to-date information, as they are more likely because of their anxiety to forget details. It is useful to have up-to-date information available of other local clinics who offer emergency contraception. If, for example, you give emergency contraception on a Friday and the client vomits and requires a second dose of pills, it is useful to give them addresses of alternative clinics if you are not available on the Saturday. It is a good idea to advertise this information in your waiting room and make it available to other staff in case they receive telephone enquiries.

The areas to be covered at counselling are summarised in Box 9.1

Box 9.1

Areas to be covered at counselling

- Record first day of last menstrual period and details of menstrual cycle length.
- Was her last menstrual period normal? Is there any possibility that she may already be pregnant? Do you need to perform a pregnancy test?
- Record the time and date of earliest UPSI; how many episodes of UPSI have there been since the first day of the last period?
- Has your client any contraindications to emergency contraception?
- What contraception was used? Is your client happy to continue with this method or does she want another method?
- Has she had emergency contraception before? Did she have any problems with it, e.g. vomiting?
- Record blood pressure.
- Does your client understand how to take the emergency contraception and know when she needs to return?
- Has your client read and been given up-to-date information about emergency contraception, and does she have contact numbers if she vomits or has a problem?

FUTURE CONTRACEPTION

If a woman is happy to continue with condoms, she needs to continue with these until she changes to another method. If, however she has been given emergency contraception and wants to start another method, she can continue with condoms until her next period and start all hormonal methods on the first day of her next period and she will be safe straightaway. Alternatively, she could "quick start" on to a hormonal method; this is an unlicensed practice which is endorsed by FSRH. You need to involve your client in the discussion about this practice and be reasonably certain that they are not already pregnant. Following LNG-EC, she could start the combined pill the next day and will need to use extra precautions for seven days; with Qlaira this will be for nine days. As her period will not be at its expected time, she should be advised to do a pregnancy test in three weeks. If the client wanted to commence the progestogen-only pill, she could also start this the following day after taking LNG-EC and should be advised to use extra precautions for two days and do a pregnancy test in three weeks.

With ulipristal acetate, the efficacy may be reduced if progestogen is quick started. This is an unlicensed practice which is endorsed by FSRH. You need to involve your client in the discussion about this practice and be reasonably certain that they are not already pregnant. If quick starting a woman onto contraception, she should be advised to take the UPA-EC and start the progestogen-only pill in five days, use extra precautions for two days and do a pregnancy test in three weeks. If she wishes to commence the combined pill, she should be advised to take the UPA-EC and start the combined pill in five days and use extra precautions for seven days, and if it is Qlaira nine days and a pregnancy test in three weeks.

Table 9.1 Quick starting contraception following LNG-EC or UPA-EC

	CHC	POP	Implant	Injectable
LNG-EC given stat	Extra precautions for 7/7 (for Qlaira 9/7), pregnancy test in 3/52	Extra precautions for 2/7, pregnancy test in 3/52	Extra precautions for 7/7, pregnancy test in 3/52	Extra precautions for 7/7, pregnancy test in 3/52
UPA-EC given stat	Start combined pill in five days. Extra precautions for 7/7 (Qlaira for 9/7), pregnancy test in 3/52	Start progestogen pill in five days. Extra precautions for 2/7, pregnancy test in 3/52	Insert implant in five days. Extra precautions for 7/7, pregnancy test in 3/52	Start injectable in five days. Extra precautions for 7/7, pregnancy test in 3/52

As quick starting is outside the product license, this will need to be discussed with the woman; however, it is endorsed by the Faculty of Sexual and Reproductive Healthcare Clinical Effectiveness Unit (FSRH, 2017b; see Table 9.1).

If a woman wishes to commence the IUS, then these can be started with the next period; alternatively, she could commence a progestogen-only pill, like Cerazette, the next day after emergency contraception, using extra precautions for two days if taking the LNG-EC or wait five days if the UPA-EC has been taken and extra precautions for two days, and return in three weeks for pregnancy test and commencement of the injectable, implant or IUS if the test is negative (Table 9.1).

Follow-up appointment

You should offer to see your client three to four weeks following post-coital contraception to check that she has had a normal menstrual period. If this is shorter or lighter than normal, a pregnancy test should be performed to exclude pregnancy. This is an excellent opportunity to encourage sexually transmitted infection screening.

PROBLEMS ENCOUNTERED WITH EMERGENCY CONTRACEPTION

- VOMITING WITH THE HORMONAL CONTRACEPTION:

  It is a good idea to try and prevent vomiting prior to it happening. Women should be encouraged to avoid taking the emergency contraception on an empty stomach. An anti-emetic like Motilium (domperidone) may be prescribed if vomiting occurs with a repeat dose of the emergency hormonal contraception. If vomiting is severe, a Cu-IUD may need to be considered.

■ PREVIOUS USE OF THE LEVONORGESTREL METHOD IN THE CYCLE AND A FURTHER EPISODE OF UNPROTECTED SEXUAL INTERCOURSE:

The levonorgestrel regimen may be given if previously used in the cycle; ulipristal acetate should not be used more than once in a cycle. It is important to check that the previous dose was taken correctly and no other UPSI has taken place other than the recent episode. If this is the case, then a Cu-IUD may be indicated if it is within five days of the earliest calculated date of ovulation.

SELF-ASSESSMENT QUESTIONS

Answers and discussion at the end of the chapter.

1 A woman with a regular cycle of 4/25 days attends requesting emergency contraception. It is 100 hours since the first episode of UPSI, and she is now on day 18 of her cycle. Can you give her emergency contraception?
2 What are the indications for emergency contraception?

THE FUTURE

Clinical guidelines are regularly updated by the Clinical Effectiveness Unit on emergency contraception by FSRH's recent guidance (FSRH, March 2017a, amended July 2023); it is important that all health professionals keep themselves up to date with changes to these.

SEXUALITY AND ANXIETIES

Men and women consulting for emergency contraception are often extremely anxious. This is exacerbated by meeting someone, often in these circumstances for the first time, to discuss intimate details of their sex life, which can make it a harrowing situation. However, if handled appropriately, it can be the beginning of a relationship that gives clients a richer knowledge and awareness of sexual health. In taking an empathetic approach with your clients which does not judge their sexual practices, you will encourage them to consult in the future.

An episode of UPSI often precipitates a change in the contraceptive method, although clients often fail to mention this. When changing methods, it is useful to ask about UPSI, as this may affect when a new method may be commenced and may also mean that emergency contraception can be discussed.

Many women perceive the hormonal method to have more risks than regularly taking the combined pill (Ziebland et al., 1996) and often accept the greater risks of an abortion by avoiding taking it. Young men and women are more likely to take the sort of risks that would require emergency contraception than older clients (Pearson et al., 1995) but are less likely to request it. This may be for a number of reasons: from lack of knowledge of its availability and awareness of its use to concern over confidentiality and fear of a hostile reception. This indicates the need to inform clients about emergency contraception – they may never need the information themselves but may inform a friend! Men should not be forgotten when educating clients about emergency contraception; increasingly, they are taking an interest and responsibility for contraception, which should be encouraged. Often, receptionists are forgotten in our zeal to educate, yet it is important that they are aware of the need of these clients to obtain immediate appointments. It is also important that they are aware of other clinics where emergency contraception is available, especially outside normal working hours, as they are most likely to receive telephone requests for this information. Giving emergency contraception can not only save a great deal of anguish over an unwanted pregnancy and abortion but is also much more cost-effective and has less risk to the health of the woman.

ANSWERS TO SELF-ASSESSMENT QUESTIONS

1   A woman with a regular cycle of 4/25 days attends requesting emergency contraception. It is 100 hours since the first episode of UPSI, and she is now on day 20 of her cycle. Can you give her emergency contraception?

   A Cu-IUD can be fitted as the UPSI is less than 5 days since the UPSI, this is the most effective emergency contraceptive method and would provide contraception until removed. She could have ulipristal acetate, which is licensed for 120 hours, or the levonorgestrel method, but this would be unlicensed, and the issue of limited data on efficacy over 96 hours would need to be discussed with her. You should advise her to return in three weeks for a pregnancy test if she has not had a normal menstrual period within that time. You should discuss future contraception, and she could quick start onto the POP or COC and use extra precautions depending on the type of hormonal emergency contraception given, or she can continue to use either condoms or abstain for contraception and commence alternative contraception with her next period.

2   What are the indications for emergency contraception?

   The indications for emergency contraception are as follows:

   ■ UPSI, e.g. condom break or misuse, diaphragm fitted incorrectly, no contraception used, missed pills, late injectable

   ■ Rape and sexual assault

   ■ Recent use of drugs with a teratogenic effect where UPSI has taken place, e.g. cytotoxic drugs, live vaccines such as yellow fever

10

MALE METHODS

The choice of contraception available to a man is limited compared with that available to a woman. Most research has been aimed at female clients because it is the woman who will become pregnant and because it is easier to stop a monthly ovulation rather than a continuous sperm process. However, with increasing education and sexual openness, more men are taking a keen interest in this area, as shown by the number of men opting for sterilisation. Health education councils and the media have tried to promote the use of the male condom in the prevention against sexually transmitted infections and HIV with limited effect; there is still the belief that "it won't happen to me," and as long as this exists, the widespread use of condoms is impeded.

- Introduction
- Coitus interruptus
- Condoms
- Male sterilisation

INTRODUCTION

Coitus interruptus is where a man withdraws his penis from the vagina before ejaculating during sexual intercourse. It is the oldest method of contraception being referred to in the Bible (Genesis 38: verse 9) and the Koran. Coitus interruptus is widely accepted and used in Muslim and Christian communities as a method of contraception. The name "coitus interruptus" is rarely used by men and women – instead it is usually referred to as withdrawal, although there are many other euphemisms such as "being careful" or "he looks after things." This can lead to misunderstanding during consultations if you are unaware of the euphemisms used for coitus interruptus, as these can vary in different areas. You may have to clarify with the client what they are practising as a method of contraception to enable you to help them during the consultation.

Explanation of the method

This is where the man withdraws his penis before ejaculating into the woman's vagina.

DOI: 10.4324/9781003484424-11

Efficacy

The efficacy of coitus interruptus is variable, but it can with careful and consistent use be as high as 96% effective in preventing pregnancy. However, the figure may be as low as 78% with less careful and committed use (Knight, 2017). Another reason why this method may fail is the presence of sperm in pre-ejaculate.

Advantages

- Easily available
- Requires no clinic appointment
- Acceptable to certain religions
- No financial cost
- Under the control of the couple

Disadvantages

- Low efficacy
- No protection against HIV and other STIs
- May inhibit enjoyment during sexual intercourse

Absolute contraindication

- Men with erectile problems such as premature ejaculation

Decision of choice

Many couples choose to use this method because of its accessibility. This may be because they have no other contraception available at the time of intercourse or because they feel that other choices are unsuitable. Coitus interruptus is often chosen as a method by couples for its religious acceptability. It may also be used initially in a new sexual relationship or where other methods seem unacceptable to the couple.

PROBLEMS ENCOUNTERED

- Pregnancy
- Sexual frustration
- Anxiety over method

Sexuality and anxieties

You may encounter anxiety by either partner. The man may feel anxious over the responsibility placed upon him to successfully withdraw his penis before ejaculation. This may reduce his enjoyment during sexual intercourse and may lead to erectile problems. The woman may experience anxiety over her partner's ability to use withdrawal and the risk of pregnancy; as a result, she may complain of loss of satisfaction during intercourse.

For many couples, this may be a highly acceptable form of contraception which is under their influence and easily reversible. They have the power to revoke their decision and have "unprotected" sexual intercourse if they wish to conceive at any time.

CONDOMS

History and introduction

Condoms were one of the first forms of contraception invented. Condoms are a highly effective method and one of the few contraceptives available to a man. They can be bought in supermarkets, petrol stations and vending machines, and are available in public male and female toilets.

Explanation of method

A condom is made from a latex sheath which is applied and covers the length of an erect penis. It is disposable and should only be used once and comes in a variety of colours and features. A condom acts as a barrier preventing sperm and ovum from meeting and pregnancy occurring. Latex-free condoms or polyurethane condoms are available for clients with latex allergies.

Efficacy

The efficacy of the condom is variable: with careful and consistent use, it can be as high as 98% or as low as 85% (FSRH, 2015c). The lower efficacy is more likely to occur in men and women who are younger and more fertile with less experience using this method. Pregnancy rates are similar for latex and non-latex condoms (FSRH, 2015c).

Disadvantages

- Perceived as messy
- Perceived as interrupting sexual intercourse
- Requires forward planning
- Loss of sensitivity
- Latex condoms cannot be used in conjunction with oil-based lubricants
- Clients with erectile problems may find applying condoms difficult

Advantages

- Under the control of the couple
- No systemic effects
- Easily available

- Protection against STIs and HIV
- May protect against cervical neoplasia

UKMEC 3 risks outweigh the benefits of using method – relative contraindication

Allergy to latex proteins
The use of condoms lubricated with nonoxynol-9 is not recommended

Range of condoms

Condoms now come in a variety of colours, flavours and shapes. Condoms must conform to the European condom standard and have the European CE mark if they are sold in Europe; in the UK, many condoms have met the British Standards Institution (BSI) specification (ISO, 4074). Condoms will carry the BSI Kitemark and the European Standard logo to ensure they have met these requirements. The use of the BSI kitemark shows that a condom complies with a recognised standard of quality and reliability. There are many flavours and shapes, including contoured, flared, plain ended, straight and ribbed.

Decision of choice

For many men and women, condoms are a convenient and easily accessible form of contraception. They allow men to share and take the responsibility for preventing pregnancy. Condoms can increase enjoyment by giving permission to men and women to touch and explore the penis. The application of a condom can be shared by either partner, creating equality in the relationship.

For many clients, choosing this method may be a spur-of-the-moment decision. It is often used initially in a sexual relationship, and these clients are usually younger. Many men and women prefer to use condoms to protect themselves against HIV.

Choosing a condom these days may be fraught with indecision for clients. How do they know which one to try? What's the difference? You are in a prime position to advise about how to use condoms and how to help your clients choose the condom most suitable for them.

There is no legal age limit requirement which restricts the sale of condoms, which gives condoms both a wide and young user age range. Many men and women stop using condoms because of complaints of loss of sensitivity. Often, change to another method is exacerbated by a user failure such as a burst condom or a condom coming off during sexual intercourse.

It is believed that one reason why men complain of loss of sensitivity with condoms is because they are too tight. Flared and contoured condoms are designed to give more space to the head of the penis, thus alleviating this problem. Contoured condoms are anatomically shaped to hug the glans so that they are less likely to slip off whilst still increasing sensitivity. Ribbed condoms are straight condoms with extra bands of latex which are designed to heighten sensitivity for a woman. Straight condoms come in designs with or without a teat (the teat is to retain ejaculate). Condoms with teats such as straight, flared or contoured should be used for internal lubrication. Internal lubrication, or "gel charging," involves putting water-soluble lubricant into the teat of the condom. As the gel liquefies around the glans, sensitivity increases; however, this has been found to be associated with an increased risk of condom slippage, and if men and woman practice this, they should be warned of this risk (FSRH, 2015c).

Condoms vary in strength. The strongest are condoms like Mates SuperSave and Durex Extra Safe, which are thicker. They are suitable for men who experience premature ejaculation or wish for other reasons to delay ejaculation. Condom breakage rates are similar for standard and thicker condoms, so there is no requirement for thicker condoms to be used for anal intercourse (FSRH, 2015c). The female condom may be used for anal intercourse if the inner ring is removed. Although male and female condoms make anal intercourse safer against STIs and HIV, they are not manufactured for this use. Condoms which are thinner are designed to increase sensitivity, but clients need to be aware of the need to apply these carefully: examples of these are Durex Thin Feel or Featherlite ultra fine. However, breakage rates are similar for standard and thicker condoms, which highlights how important it is to teach condom application correctly.

It is no longer recommended that condoms contain the spermicide nonoxynol-9, which may increase local irritation and increase transmission of STIs and HIV transmission (FSRH, 2015c). If a partner complains of local irritation to a condom, then a condom using a non-spermicidal lubricant should be used once genitourinary infections have been excluded.

Flavoured condoms are suitable for oral intercourse and come in a variety of flavours and colours. Condoms are available in discrete packaging aimed at different age groups.

Loss of efficacy of the condom

Various preparations affect the efficacy of the condom. Oil-based preparations should not be used with latex-containing condoms, as they damage the latex rubber; these include lipstick, body oils, massage oils, baby oils butter, ice cream and Vaseline. Vaginal and topical preparations should not be used with latex, as they may cause damage; these include econazole, miconazole, isoconazole, fenticonazole and clotrimazole.

Teaching how to use a condom

Teaching clients how to use and apply a condom requires little time yet may prevent user failure. Research indicates that condom breakages are more common in young and inexperienced clients (Sparrow & Lavill, 1994). Other condom failures were where the condom slipped off inside the vagina following loss of erection after sexual intercourse. Condom mishaps are most likely to occur at the beginning of a relationship (UK Family Planning Research Network, 1993) and decrease as the relationship continues. This means that new and transient relationships are most at risk of unprotected sexual intercourse.

All this information shows how important it is to teach clients how to use condoms. When teaching your clients, it is helpful to show how to apply a condom using a condom demonstrator. Encourage your client to check that the condom packet has not expired and has the BSI Kitemark and CE logo. When opening the condom packet, clients should push the condom out of the way to avoid tearing; the condom packet should then be squeezed helping the condom to slip out. A condom should be applied before the penis comes into contact with the vulva. The condom should be placed on the erect penis and unrolled carefully along the whole length of it. Using their other hand, the client should squeeze the condom at the head of the penis to expel any air. Once ejaculation has taken place, the penis should be withdrawn, holding the condom onto the base of the penis to ensure that it is not left in the vagina. Condoms should only be used once and disposed of carefully.

You should discuss with your client the loss of efficacy caused by oil-based lubricants and give up-to-date information on condoms. As all methods of contraception have a failure rate, it is important to discuss emergency contraception and post-exposure prophylaxis after sexual exposure (PEPSE) to HIV. There are still large gaps in men's and women's knowledge on emergency contraception, so this is a good time to correct misconceptions.

ACTIVITY

Practise applying condoms with either a condom demonstrator or your fingers. Do you know what condoms are available where you work?

PROBLEMS ENCOUNTERED

There are a number of accidents that can be encountered whilst using condoms.

■ THE CONDOM BURST OR SPLIT DURING SEXUAL INTERCOURSE:
    This is usually because the client has either put the condom on inside out or not released any air, or the condom has come into contact with a fat-soluble product, e.g. baby oil which caused the condom to break.
■ THE CONDOM SLIPPED OFF DURING INTERCOURSE OR REMAINED INSIDE THE VAGINA WHEN THE PENIS WAS REMOVED FOLLOWING INTERCOURSE:
    This usually happens when a man loses his erection and fails to hold onto the condom when he removes his penis from the vagina, leaving the condom inside the vagina. The condom can also slip off when applied inside out.
■ THE CONDOM WAS RIPPED WHILST IT WAS APPLIED:
    This can be due to ragged nails or rings, and a new condom should be applied if this happens.
■ DIFFICULTIES APPLYING THE CONDOM – "IT'S TOO SMALL OR TOO BIG":
    Condoms can now be bought to accommodate different sizes of penis. All condoms can expand, so they should not be too small. However, Mates now makes condoms in contoured and flared shapes; flared are suitable for men who complain that the condom is too small and contoured for men who find condoms too big, like Mates Conform. EXS also make a condom called Snug Fit for men who want smaller-sized condoms.

■ LOSS OF THE SENSITIVITY:
Condoms which are plain ended and thin will help increase sensitivity. Men complain of loss of sensitivity because the condom is too tight; flared condoms may help alleviate this problem.

Case history

A 33-year-old married woman consulted concerned that she had a condom left inside her vagina. The condom was found and removed from the vagina. During the session, the nurse asked whether emergency contraception was wanted, and whether the woman was happy with her method of contraception.

The woman was trying to conceive but explained that the condom was from another partner, and she would therefore want emergency contraception. As she has already had unprotected sexual intercourse with her regular partner with whom she was trying to conceive throughout her cycle, and was now beyond the limits for emergency contraception, this was contraindicated. The risks of this episode of unprotected sexual intercourse were discussed in relation to pregnancy and genitourinary infection. A pregnancy test was performed which was negative and a further test was arranged for a week's time when the client's next period was due.

SELF-ASSESSMENT QUESTIONS

Answers and discussion at the end of the chapter.

1   What sort of condom would you recommend for anal intercourse?
2   Name ten products which will cause condoms to burst.

Sexuality and anxieties

Men and women often consult following accidents with condoms for emergency contraception. New relationships appear to be the riskiest time for condom breakages (UK Family Planning Research Network, 1993). However, research with commercial sex workers in the United States (Albert et al., 1995) suggests that regular condom use leads to the development of techniques which reduce breakage and slippage of condoms. When clients consult for emergency contraception following a condom breakage, this is a prime opportunity to discuss condom technique and alleviate any future problems. Many men and women use a condom breakage as their reason for requiring emergency contraception when in fact they have had unprotected sexual intercourse which they feel will be disapproved of by professionals. This makes it difficult to obtain accurate statistics for condom use and breakage.

Condoms give a man the opportunity to take part in contraception; they are often used at some point in a relationship and have the advantage of taking care of the "mess." However, for some women, this may be the very reason why they dislike condoms; the "mess" or ejaculate may be warm and exciting.

Condoms can give a woman permission to touch her partner's penis; she can use a condom as part of a safe form of foreplay by applying it herself or together with her partner. This can give couples the opportunity to talk about their sexual needs and desires.

MALE STERILISATION

History and introduction

Male sterilisation has become a popular choice of permanent contraception for many couples; the surgical procedure is known as a vasectomy.

Explanation of the method

A vasectomy involves cutting the vas deferens, which is the tube that transports sperm from the epididymis in the testes to the seminal vesicles. By cutting the vas deferens, sperm is unable to be ejaculated, and a man will become infertile once the vas deferens is clear of sperm, which takes about three months.

Efficacy

A vasectomy is a highly effective form of contraception. Its immediate failure rate is 1 in 2,000 (FSRH, 2014a).

Disadvantages

- Alternative contraception is required until two consecutive clear sperm counts are obtained
- Surgical procedure required
- Local or general anaesthesia required
- Not easily reversible

Advantages

- Permanent method
- High efficacy
- Removal of anxiety of unplanned pregnancy
- Safe and simple procedure

Absolute contraindications

- Serious physical disability
- Urological problems
- Relationship problems
- Indecision by either partner

Range of method

During a vasectomy, the vas deferens will be cut and either cautery or a ligature will be applied. Part of the incised vas deferens may be sent to pathology to confirm that the correct tube has been cut. Each end of the vas deferens will be buried in separate tissue layers to prevent them from re-joining (see Figure 10.1). Research comparing traditional surgery for vasectomies with electrocautery non-scalpel vasectomy techniques found that men experienced less pain and bleeding from the wound with this method (Black, 2003); the non-scalpel method is now the recommended choice for a vasectomy surgery (RCOG, 2004; FSRH, 2014a).

Side effects

- Infection
- Haematoma
- Sperm granuloma

Counselling a couple for a vasectomy

Vasectomy counselling is preferably performed with both partners, as this is a decision which will permanently affect both parties. As this is a permanent method of contraception, the couple should be sure of their decision and aware that this is very difficult to reverse. During counselling, couples are often asked to consider certain scenarios, e.g. how they would feel if their partner died, would they want to have more? If they have not had children, is there a likelihood they will change their mind? Sometimes clients have not considered

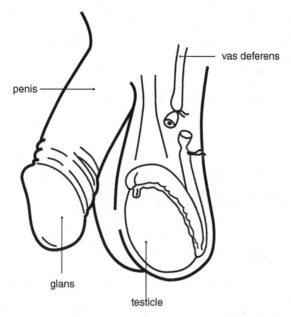

Figure 10.1 Male sterilisation (vasectomy).

major life events and their effects, and during counselling decide to delay such a permanent decision.

Men are often concerned about their ability to maintain erections and have sexual intercourse following a vasectomy. You can advise your clients that a vasectomy does not affect libido or erections, and their ejaculate will look the same except it will no longer contain sperm, which is not detectable to the human eye.

It is important that your client continues to use an effective form of contraception, as it may cause considerable distress if a client has a vasectomy and then finds his partner is pregnant. Contraception will be required for about three months following a vasectomy. Once consecutive negative sperm counts have been obtained, then the use of another form of contraception may be ceased.

There has been concern over an increased incidence of testicular (West, 1992) and prostate cancer (Giovannucci et al., 1993a, 1993b) in men who have had a vasectomy. At the moment, there is no increased link between cancer of the prostate or testes and vasectomies (RCOG, 2004; FSRH, 2014a). It may be that men who have had a vasectomy are more aware and consult earlier if they notice a problem (Howards & Peterson, 1993). Smoking increases the risk of all cancers, including testicular and prostate cancer. Cancer of the prostate is a disease found in older men; 90% of all deaths from cancer of the prostate occur after the age of 65.

Vasectomies can fail even after negative sperm counts, and it is important to discuss this with your client beforehand (Brahams, 1995). This is thought to be due to re-canalisation of the vas deferens.

Procedure

A vasectomy may be performed under local or general anaesthetic. One or two incisions are performed on each scrotum so that the vas deferens may be located, excised and ligated.

Post vasectomy

Men should be encouraged to take things gently, as this will reduce the risk of bruising. They should wear scrotal support and avoid heavy lifting, strenuous exercise and sexual intercourse for a week postoperatively. Pain may be eased by the use of ice packs and analgesia; frozen peas are suitable for this purpose, as they mould around the area well, reducing swelling and pain. A follow-up study of men who had had a vasectomy (Canter & Goldthorpe, 1995) found that the median time to full recovery after the operation was seven days. Many clients do not allow enough time for full recovery, which increases their chances of getting postoperative complications.

A man should complete a sperm test to ensure the surgery has been successful and semen analysis is clear of sperm at 12 weeks post-surgery (FSRH, 2024b). Semen analysis will need to be repeated at four to six weeks if the sample shows more than 100,000 mL non-motile sperm or motile sperm (FSRH, 2024b). If the semen analysis is clear of sperm, then the man will be advised he can stop using another form of contraception. It takes about three months for a man's ejaculate to clear of sperm.

Following a vasectomy, a man should watch for any signs of infection, haematoma and sperm granuloma. Any signs of rising temperature and/or pain or swelling around the testes may indicate infection, which will need to be treated with antibiotics. A haematoma is likely to happen if a client has not given himself enough time to recuperate; it should be treated with ice packs, analgesia and rest. A sperm granuloma can cause pain and localised swelling but can also be asymptomatic; it occurs when sperm leaks into the surrounding tissue where the vas deferens was excised and may need further excision.

Reversal of vasectomy

Reversal is often requested when a man has commenced a new relationship and wishes to have children. Reversal of a vasectomy is easier to perform than reversal of a female sterilisation. However, success is variable and can be between 52% and 82% in achieving a pregnancy (RCOG, 2004); this may be higher in skilled hands and may be lower if the operation was performed more than ten years ago. When reversing a vasectomy, the vas deferens is re-anastomosed, which may be successful, but there is a risk that anti-sperm antibodies will develop and cause the sperm count to be low, making pregnancy difficult to achieve.

SELF-ASSESSMENT QUESTIONS

Answers and discussion at the end of the chapter.

3 Roughly how long does it take for a man to achieve a negative sperm count following a vasectomy?
4 What advantages do you think a vasectomy has over female sterilisation?
5 What anxieties may a man have over a vasectomy?

ACTIVITY

Do you know what facilities are available locally for men requesting a vasectomy? Is there a waiting list? What are your clients told about aftercare? Are you giving the same information?

Sexuality and anxieties

Vasectomies have become more fashionable in recent times; this coincides with the "sharing, caring image" of "new men." However, sometimes it can be used as an emotional weapon – women may say, "It's his turn to do something now," which may cause conflict in the future in their relationship. There can be an element of self-sacrifice and martyrdom about the decision, which is why meeting both parties at the counselling session may help to bring this into open discussion.

A vasectomy may be chosen following completion of a family but also may be the result of an unplanned pregnancy, which may scare a couple into deciding.

After a vasectomy, some men may experience signs of grief over their loss of fertility and sexuality. This will depend on how the man feels about his decision; if he feels forced or coerced into the decision, then he may feel anger and sadness over his loss. Some men see a vasectomy as tantamount to castration and have anxieties that their ability to function as a man will be impaired permanently. Many men see a vasectomy as their opportunity to do something, especially after their partner has had children. This can cement their relationship and bring them closer, reducing anxiety over further pregnancy.

ANSWERS TO SELF-ASSESSMENT QUESTIONS

1   What sort of condom would you recommend for anal intercourse?

Although condoms are not manufactured for anal intercourse, there are no recommendations for the type of condom to use for anal intercourse. Condom breakage rates are similar for standard and thicker condom. A water-based lubricant should be used in conjunction with a condom for anal intercourse to reduce breakage.

2   Name ten products which will cause condoms to burst.

Oil-based preparations should not be used with latex-containing condoms as they damage the latex rubber; these include lipstick, body oils, massage oils, baby oils butter, ice cream and Vaseline. Vaginal and topical preparation should not be used with latex, as they may cause damage; these include econazole, miconazole, isoconazole, fenticonazole and clotrimazole.

3   Roughly, how long does it take for a man to achieve a negative sperm count following a vasectomy?

It takes roughly three months for a man to achieve a negative sperm count, and he can consider it safe to have sexual intercourse when he has had two consecutive negative sperm counts.

4   What advantages do you think a vasectomy has over female sterilisation?

A vasectomy can easily be performed under local anaesthetic, whilst the majority of female sterilisations are performed under general anaesthetic. Anatomically, the scrotum and vas deferens are easy to locate, whilst with a woman locating the fallopian tubes is harder, as they are under muscle and fat layers. This is why women may be in hospital for longer, whilst a man may go home following the procedure.

5   What anxieties may a man have over a vasectomy?

Men have anxieties over their ability to achieve an orgasm, maintain an erection and changes in their ejaculate. Most of their anxieties surround myths about vasectomy, which include impotence and sexual dysfunction. They may also have anxieties over prostate and testicular cancer. Some men may have anxieties about the procedure and fears about what may happen.

11

FEMALE BARRIER METHODS

THE DIAPHRAGM

Introduction

Contraception not only gives women protection against pregnancy but also gives women power over their bodies. The diaphragm gives women the opportunity to understand and get to know their bodies. Whilst it is not widely used, many women would like to use it but find it difficult to find a healthcare professional who has the skills to teach it. The diaphragm is often used by women who are spacing pregnancies.

Explanation of method

The diaphragm is a dome made of silicone which is inserted into the vagina. It covers the cervix, acting as a barrier to sperm and therefore helping to prevent pregnancy.

Efficacy

With careful and consistent use, the diaphragm is 92%–96% effective when used with a spermicide in preventing pregnancy in the first year. However, with typical use, where a woman does not use the diaphragm carefully and consistently, the efficacy is 82%–90%; this is when used with spermicide (Bounds, 1994).

Failure rates for the diaphragm depend on how effectively the woman uses it. Does she use the diaphragm for every episode of sexual intercourse? Is her cervix covered during each episode? Is she using her diaphragm according to guidelines? Other factors which influence the failure rate of all methods are a woman's age and how often she is having sexual intercourse. For example, if a woman is aged 40 and uses a diaphragm as a contraceptive, she is less fertile than a woman aged 25, so a diaphragm is a more effective contraceptive for her.

The use of a spermicide with the diaphragm is currently recommended (FSRH, 2015c). The only study which compared the diaphragm with and without spermicide (Bounds et al., 1995) did not give significant results for the use of a diaphragm being effective if used alone. Until research proves that a diaphragm is as effective without spermicide as it is with spermicide, current guidelines recommend that you teach your client to continue to use the diaphragm with a spermicide.

DOI: 10.4324/9781003484424-12

Disadvantages

■ Requires motivation
■ Needs to be used carefully and consistently for optimum efficacy
■ Needs to be used with a spermicide which may be perceived as messy
■ May increase the risk of cystitis and urinary tract infections
■ No protection against HIV

Advantages

■ Under the control of the woman
■ May give some protection against cervical cancer and sexually transmitted diseases
■ No systemic side effects
■ Provides vaginal lubrication
■ Can be used during menstruation
■ Gives a woman permission to touch and explore her body

UKMEC 4 – NONE

UKMEC 3 risks outweigh the benefits of using method – relative contraindications

■ Allergy to rubber or spermicide
■ Pregnancy
■ Undiagnosed genital tract bleeding should be investigated and treated first
■ Poor vaginal muscle tone or prolapse
■ Congenital abnormality such as two cervices or septal wall defects (where the vagina is separated into two by a wall)
■ Present vaginal, cervical or pelvic infection should be investigated and treated first
■ Past history of toxic shock syndrome
■ HIV – women who are HIV positive or at high risk of HIV infection
■ Use of spermicides containing nonoxynol-9 is associated with genital lesions and may increase the risk of acquiring HIV or other infections

Side effects

■ Urinary tract infection
■ Toxic shock syndrome – diaphragms and caps should not be left in situ for longer than recommended by the manufacturer or used during menstruation, as they are associated with an increased risk
■ Vaginal irritation

Range of method

There are two main types of diaphragms. Ortho Johnson was the maker of the All-Flex diaphragm; however, production ceased in 2014. Currently, Milex manufactures the Omniflex and arcing diaphragms, which retail at £49.85 each. However, a diaphragm is free on the NHS and should be fitted by a trained nurse or doctor.

Omniflex coil spring diaphragm

The Omniflex diaphragm has a wide seal rim which can be folded in any direction and has a coiled spring in the rim; it is available in sizes 60–90 mm (rising in steps of 5 mm) and is made of silicone. This type of diaphragm is suitable for all women.

Arcing spring diaphragm

This type of diaphragm is available in sizes 60–90 mm (rising in steps of 5 mm) and is made of silicone. This type of diaphragm is suitable for women with a posterior positioned cervix, or where a woman has difficulty feeling her cervix.

Decision of choice

The decision of the type of diaphragm you fit your client will depend on a vaginal examination. You will need to assess the vagina and cervix to exclude infection, poor muscle tone and prolapse. When examining your client to estimate the size of diaphragm required, you should measure the distance from the posterior fornix (the area immediately behind the cervix) to the symphysis pubis (the bone in front of the bladder) with your fingers (Figure 11.1).

The measurement on your fingers corresponds to the size of diaphragm required for your client (Figure 11.2). With practice you will find that this is not difficult; it can be useful beforehand to measure your fingers to see where a diaphragm measures on your fingers. The diaphragm should be fitted now to check that the

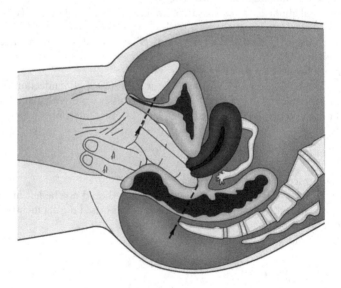

Figure 11.1 Estimating the size of the diaphragm to be fitted.

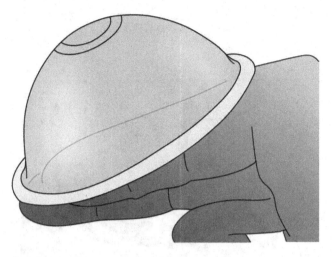

Figure 11.2 Size of diaphragm on hand.

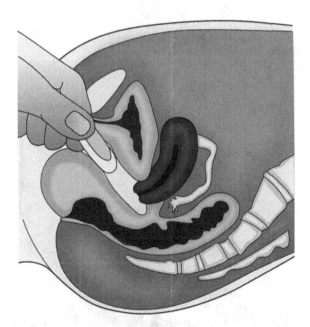

Figure 11.3 Diaphragm being inserted.

correct size has been chosen (Figures 11.3 and 11.4). The diaphragm should cover the cervix and sit tucked up behind the symphysis pubis. If it protrudes into the introitus, then the diaphragm is either too large (Figure 11.5) or fitted incorrectly. If there is a gap of a finger or more, then the diaphragm is too small (Figure 11.6). Your client should be unable to feel the diaphragm *in situ* if fitted correctly.

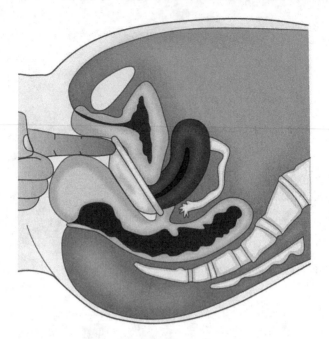

Figure 11.4 Checking the position of the diaphragm.

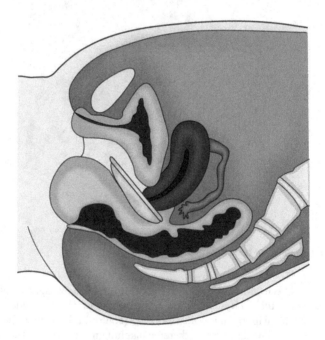

Figure 11.5 Diaphragm too large.

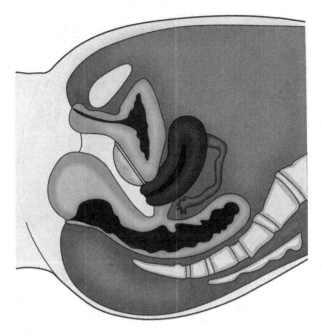

Figure 11.6 Diaphragm too small.

How to teach a diaphragm fitting

This can feel like a very threatening and embarrassing situation to your client, so it is important that your examination room is quiet, private and free from interruptions. This consultation can take some time, so allow at least half an hour; you will both feel more at ease if time is not an issue. Usually, a diaphragm-fitting teaching session is spread over two consultations. The first visit includes initial fitting and teaching the client to locate her cervix and remove and fit the diaphragm. The second consultation includes teaching spermicidal application. Although this can be done at either visit, it is useful to have a second consultation to solve any problems. The more comfortable your client feels, the more at ease she will be in the situation and the more likely she is to succeed. Before examining your client, you should show her a diaphragm and, using diagrams or a teaching model, show her how the diaphragm sits inside the vagina. Some women find this slightly difficult to understand at first, and how you approach this will vary with each client. Try and find out how much she knows and build upon this. Remember, the majority of women may have never felt their cervix or have thought much about its significance. Discuss how you are going to teach your client to fit her diaphragm; this will help her feel more comfortable with the situation.

Once you have estimated the correct size of diaphragm and it is in situ, your client should be taught to feel inside her vagina and feel the position of the diaphragm and cervix. It is helpful if you wear a pair of gloves during this part of the consultation in case you need to help her by holding the diaphragm at some point. To teach your client, she should be encouraged to wash her hands and either squat or put one foot on a chair. She should then feel inside her vagina so that she can understand how the diaphragm sits (Figure 11.7). You will now need

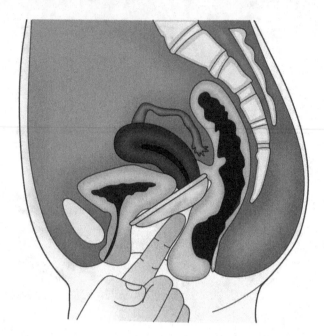

Figure 11.7 Checking a diaphragm covering the cervix (standing position).

her to feel inside her vagina. It is helpful if you give your client an idea of where her cervix is positioned and what it feels like. The cervix has been described as a fleshy lump feeling like the end of your nose. It is important that she is able to locate her cervix so that she is aware of it being covered by the diaphragm to ensure efficacy.

When your client is able to locate her cervix, ask her to remove her diaphragm by putting her index finger over the anterior rim of the diaphragm and pulling downwards (Figure 11.8). The diaphragm should slip easily out. If she finds this difficult ask her to bear downwards, making removal easier. You may want to take the diaphragm and rinse it for your client so that it does not become too slippery initially for her to fit. She can insert the diaphragm by squeezing it together firmly with one hand or by using her thumb and second index finger to squeeze it together whilst her first index finger remains inside the diaphragm, giving more control over it. The diaphragm should then be inserted into the vagina as far as it will go, pushing the anterior rim of the diaphragm underneath the ledge of the symphysis pubis. Encourage your client to check that her cervix is covered, and that she feels that the diaphragm is fitted correctly. Next check by examination that your client has fitted her diaphragm correctly.

Once your client is able to locate her cervix, fit and remove her diaphragm, she is able to practise using it. Usually, a second consultation is made about a week later. This allows your client time to practise, whilst she uses another form of contraception to avoid pregnancy. During this time, she should sleep with the diaphragm *in situ*, open her bowels, have sexual intercourse and practise removing and fitting her diaphragm so that if she has any problems, these can be discussed and solved. Occasionally, it may be necessary to combine both visits into one.

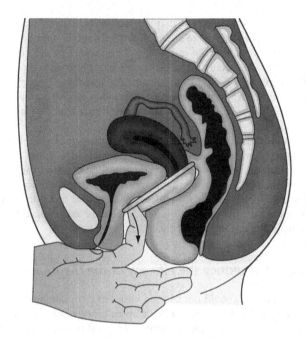

Figure 11.8 Client removing a diaphragm (standing position).

At the next visit, you should advise your client to come with her diaphragm already in place. By doing this, you will be able to check that she is able to fit her diaphragm correctly. This is a good time to revise care of the diaphragm, how to use spermicide and how long the diaphragm should be left in situ. All this information should be backed up with the appropriate leaflets, details of when your client should consult early and when a routine consultation should be carried out.

You should weigh your client at both consultations and advise her that if her weight fluctuates by 3 kg either way, she will need to have her diaphragm checked and may require a smaller or larger diaphragm to be fitted.

The success of these consultations is very much down to the approach you give the session. If you are teaching your client to locate her cervix and she is having difficulty, if she is using a squatting position, you may find that communication between you both is improved if you assume a squatting position so that you are both at the same eye level. Given time and an empathetic approach, your client will gain confidence to succeed. Often, clients will have problems fitting the diaphragm and locating their cervix and may need longer at the initial consultation. Sometimes, depending on the client, you may find giving her some time by herself helpful if she feels hampered by the situation. It is important to assess each client individually; some women may require more privacy than others.

Use of the diaphragm

If your client gets into the habit of putting her diaphragm in regularly at the time she is most likely to have sexual intercourse, then she is less likely to forget to put it in prior to intercourse. The diaphragm should be fitted with two 2 cm strips of spermicidal gel on both sides of the diaphragm. This will give contraceptive protection for three hours. After three hours, if no sexual intercourse has taken place, more spermicide will need to be inserted, e.g. pessary. However, if sexual intercourse has taken place, and further intercourse is likely later than three hours after insertion, the diaphragm should be left *in situ* and additional spermicide inserted into the vagina five to ten minutes prior to intercourse to give additional cover.

The diaphragm should be left *in situ* for six hours after the last episode of sexual intercourse.

Lastly, it is important to cover care of the diaphragm. It should be washed with mild soap and water and dried. Talcum powders, detergents and perfumes should be avoided, as these will affect the natural flora in the vagina. The diaphragm should be bent back into shape and kept in its case following use. The diaphragm should be kept away from direct sunlight and radiators, as these may cause the diaphragm to perish. Your client should be encouraged to check her diaphragm for holes, as these will reduce its effectiveness.

Preparations that reduce the efficacy of the diaphragm

Oil-based preparations should not be used with latex-containing diaphragms, as they damage the latex rubber; these include lipstick, body oils, massage oils, baby oils butter, ice cream and Vaseline. Vaginal and topical preparation should not be used with latex, as they may cause damage; these include econazole, miconazole, isoconazole, fenticonazole and clotrimazole.

Subsequent visits

You should see your client routinely every six months to check that the diaphragm is being fitted correctly by her and to review weight. The diaphragm should be renewed every year.

You should advise your client to return earlier if any of the following happens:

- Her weight varies by 3 kg.
- Her diaphragm deteriorates, has a hole, etc.
- The diaphragm becomes uncomfortable.
- Pregnancy. The diaphragm should be checked following any pregnancy, e.g. miscarriage, abortion and birth.
- She has a vaginal infection. A new diaphragm should be fitted once the infection has been investigated and treated to prevent re-infection.

SELF-ASSESSMENT QUESTIONS

Answers and discussion at the end of the chapter.

1 Which preparations should not be used with a diaphragm?
2 How would you help a client who is unable to locate her cervix?
3 For which clients would an arcing diaphragm be appropriate?

PROBLEMS ENCOUNTERED

The following are some problems you may encounter during your consultation.

■ YOUR CLIENT IS UNABLE TO LOCATE HER CERVIX:
This can be because your client lacks confidence and needs more time. Try asking her to assume a different position, i.e. squatting or placing a foot on a chair. Sometimes you may meet a client who has regularly been using a diaphragm but has never been taught to locate her cervix.
If your client's cervix is very posterior, then it will be easier for her if you fit an arcing diaphragm. An arcing diaphragm has a spring which causes the diaphragm to fall naturally to the posterior part of the vagina.
■ THE DIAPHRAGM DOES NOT COVER YOUR CLIENT'S CERVIX:
This can be because the diaphragm is too small, and she needs a larger-sized diaphragm or because her cervix is posterior, and an arcing diaphragm is more suitable.
■ YOUR CLIENT IS UNABLE TO REMOVE HER DIAPHRAGM:
Ask your client to bear downwards as this usually helps with removal. Remind her that the diaphragm cannot get lost. If she cannot remove it at that time, then she should not panic but leave removal until she is more relaxed.
■ YOUR CLIENT COMPLAINS THAT HER PARTNER CAN FEEL THE DIAPHRAGM:
If your client complains that her partner can feel the diaphragm, check that the diaphragm is the correct size, and she is fitting it correctly.
■ YOUR CLIENT COMPLAINS OF RECURRENT CYSTITIS:
If your client complains of recurrent cystitis, encourage her to empty her bladder before having sexual intercourse. You should also check her diaphragm; it may be an incorrect size. If she has a flat spring diaphragm, then changing her diaphragm to a coiled spring, which is softer, will help. Research has shown that women using a diaphragm were two to three times more likely to be referred with a urinary tract infection than women not using a diaphragm (Vessey, 1988), so women experiencing recurrent urine tract infections may need to review their method of contraception.

THE FEMCAP

The FemCap is the only cervical cap licensed in the UK and costs £30.80; it is designed to conform to the natural shape of the cervix, and the brim around it serves to create a seal around the vaginal wall, stopping sperm from entering the vagina. It is made of medical-grade silicone rubber and has a strap to aid removal and can be left *in situ* for 48 hours. The FemCap should be left *in situ* eight hours after sexual intercourse. There are three sizes: the smallest 22 mm is intended for nulliparous women, the 26 mm size is suitable for women who have been pregnant but not had a vaginal delivery and the largest size is 30 mm, suitable for women who have had a vaginal delivery. Research has found the FemCap to be 86.5% effective in preventing pregnancy; if used carefully and consistently, it may be 98% effective in preventing pregnancy; what is certain is that the efficacy is no worse than the diaphragm (American Health Consultants, 2000).

Sexuality and anxieties

A client who chooses to use a diaphragm and is successful with it can find the diaphragm gives her permission to investigate her vagina, allowing her to touch areas that may have seemed forbidden. Often, women have little or no knowledge of this area of their body and have built up their own ideas about their vagina. Not only can a diaphragm act as a contraceptive, but it can also educate and illuminate a hidden area.

You may find that your client complains that her diaphragm is "messy." This may be due to real problems with a type of spermicide, but often, there is an underlying problem. A client who complains that her diaphragm is messy may feel that sexual intercourse is messy. Some women have fantasies about their vagina – they feel that it is a clean, sterile area and forget that it produces its own natural discharge. They find sperm messy, and as a result of these feelings, there may be a problem with sexual intercourse. Given time and awareness of the feelings that the client is transferring, you will find that she may talk about her anxieties. However, sometimes clients are not ready or able to look at their feelings but may do so in the future.

Clients may panic if they are unable to remove their diaphragm. Behind this may lie the image that the diaphragm has disappeared into the midst of nowhere. Through lack of knowledge, men and women can create very strong images of their bodies which can be frightening and strange.

A woman who chooses the diaphragm may do so because of its lower efficacy compared to other methods. She may have a subconscious desire to become pregnant or may actively use the method to become pregnant without letting her partner know.

THE FEMALE CONDOM

Introduction and history

The female condom is available over the counter to all women and has helped to increase the choices open to women.

Explanation of the method

The female condom is made of lubricated polyurethane. It is 170 mm in length and has an outer ring and an inner ring. The inner ring, which is situated at the closed end of the condom, is used to aid insertion. The outer ring is situated at the open end of the condom and lies flat against the vulva. The female condom prevents sperm from entering the vagina by acting as a barrier.

Efficacy

The female condom is 95% effective in preventing pregnancy (FSRH, 2015c).

Disadvantages

- Is perceived as noisy
- Requires motivation
- May be perceived as interrupting sexual intercourse

Advantages

- Is under the control of the woman
- Protects against sexually transmitted infections and HIV
- Can be used in conjunction with oil-based products
- Has no systemic side effects

Range of method

There is one female condom available in the UK.

How to teach the use of the female condom

You should advise your client to insert the female condom by squeezing the smaller ring at the closed end of the condom between her thumb and index finger. She should then insert the ring into the vagina as far as she can and insert her finger into the condom. This will push the condom upwards into the vagina and allow the outer ring to lie flat against the vulva. The inner ring does not need to lie over the cervix and should be left *in situ*.

The woman's partner should insert his penis into the condom, with the outer ring lying flat against the vulva. Care should be taken that the penis is not inserted between the condom and the vagina. Once ejaculation has taken place, the outer ring should be twisted so that the ejaculate is retained in the female condom and gently pulled out of the vagina. The female condom should be disposed of in a rubbish bin; it cannot be flushed down a toilet.

1 The small ring which lies within the closed end of the condom helps to insert the female condom much like a tampon and holds the condom in place in the vagina. To insert, firmly hold the small ring between the thumb and middle finger.
2 Find a comfortable position, either lying down, sitting with the knees apart or standing with one foot up on a chair. Insert the squeezed ring into the vagina, pushing it inside as far as possible.
3 Put a finger inside the condom and push the small ring inside as far as it can go, like a tampon. Most women do not feel the inner ring once the female condom is inserted. Some may find that insertion is fully completed by the penis when it enters the vagina. There is no need for the female condom to be fitted over the cervix.
4 It is normal for part of the condom to hang outside the body. The outer ring helps keep the condom in place and will lie flat against the body when the penis is inside the condom. Most couples do not feel the outer ring during use.

5 The penis should be guided inside the condom. As long as the penis remains inside the sheath and the outer ring remains outside the body, the female condom is working.

6 To remove, twist the outer ring to contain the semen and gently pull the female condom out. The female condom must be removed before the risk of spilling any ejaculate, immediately after loss of erection.

Like male condoms, the female condom can be used only once and must not be flushed down the toilet.

All teaching should be supported by relevant written information.

Counselling

The female condom is suitable for women with a latex allergy. It is also ideal for women who are concerned about HIV and sexually transmitted infections. It feels stronger and more durable than a male condom and is not affected by oil-based lubricants.

Women can insert the female condom prior to sexual intercourse. They will find that it will stay *in situ* if they move around as long as they have fitted it correctly. Some women have mistakenly removed the inner ring of the condom which helps keep the condom in position.

Although research (Bounds et al., 1992a) has shown that the female condom is not aesthetically pleasing to many women and their partners, a number of positive features were highlighted. These included that the female condom rarely splits and that there was less loss of sensitivity experienced by men compared with the male condom.

PROBLEMS ENCOUNTERED

■ PENIS INSERTED OUTSIDE THE FEMALE CONDOM:
Clients should be advised to insert the penis carefully and be aware of this problem and informed about emergency contraception.

■ FEMALE CONDOM REMOVED AS THE PENIS IS WITHDRAWN:
Clients should be encouraged to hold onto the outside ring as the penis is withdrawn.

■ CLIENT COMPLAINS OF NOISE:
Some women have complained about a rustling noise; others however have commented that they do not mind the sound. The use of additional spermicide or lubrication may help to reduce this problem, but this may make the condom more slippery.

SELF-ASSESSMENT QUESTIONS

Answers and discussion at the end of the chapter.

4 What advantages do you think the female condom has that would appeal to a woman?

Sexuality and anxieties

The female condom may seem unappealing to some women because of its appearance, or the "rustling sound" made. However, in a relationship that is open and understanding, this method may be a very acceptable choice. Research (Bounds et al., 1992a) has shown that a small proportion of couples may prefer this method over the male condom, as they found sexual intercourse more enjoyable. Other couples have experienced less loss of sensitivity with the female condom.

In another study where the female condom's acceptability and experience were researched (Ford & Mathie, 1993), clients commented that they liked the "lack of mess." Some women encouraged their partners to insert the condom, which they found enjoyable. Other women found the insertion of the female condom embarrassing and awkward. It was also noted that, like all methods, men and women found insertion easier with prolonged use.

SPERMICIDES

Introduction and history

Spermicides are usually used with another method of contraception such as the diaphragm and condom.

Explanation of the method

Spermicides inactivate sperm by causing changes in the cell membrane of the spermatozoa.

Efficacy

There is little information on the efficacy of spermicides used on their own. They are believed to be of only a moderate efficacy, which is why it is recommended that they are used in conjunction with another form of contraception.

Disadvantages

- Perceived as messy
- Local allergic reaction
- Only of moderate contraceptive efficacy

Advantages

- Provides lubrication
- Is easily available
- May provide protection against sexually transmitted infections and HIV
- Can be used in conjunction with the barrier methods of contraception

Absolute contraindication

■ Allergic reaction to spermicides

Range of method

Spermicides are available in the form of Gygel.

Side effect

■ Local irritation

Counselling

There is no evidence that condoms lubricated with spermicides increase efficacy, and the addition of spermicide to condoms during vaginal sex is not recommended, as it can increase condom slippage (FSRH, 2015c). Nonoxynol-9 has been demonstrated in laboratory research to be effective *in vitro* against HIV (Chantler, 1992). However, it has been found to increase the risk of genital lesions in the rectum and vagina which may increase HIV transmission. Nonoxynol-9 use is therefore not recommended with condoms (FSRH, 2015c).

ANSWERS TO SELF-ASSESSMENT QUESTIONS

1 Which preparations should not be used with a diaphragm?

The following preparations should not be used with a diaphragm, as they damage the latex rubber: lipstick, body oils, massage oils, baby oils butter, ice cream, Vaseline. Vaginal and topical preparation should not be used with latex, as they may cause damage; these include econazole, miconazole, isoconazole, fenticonazole and clotrimazole.

2 How would you help a client who is unable to locate her cervix?

If a client is unable to locate her cervix, then try getting her to assume a different position to feel her cervix, like squatting or with a foot on a chair. If your client is happy, her partner could check that her cervix is covered.

3 For which clients would an arcing diaphragm be appropriate?

An arcing diaphragm is suitable for a woman with a posterior cervix, or for someone who is having problems locating her cervix or fitting her diaphragm.

4 What advantages do you think the female condom has that would appeal to a woman?

The female condom has many advantages that appeal to women. Women who have anxiety over sexually transmitted infections and HIV because their partner has sexual intercourse outside the relationship have commented that they prefer this method because it gives them control over contraception combined with safer sex. The female condom may appeal to women who suffer from recurrences of genital herpes. It also gives a wider choice for sex workers practising safer sex.

The female condom may appeal to women who are physically disabled, as it has no systemic effects and can be inserted by her partner as part of foreplay. Any woman or her partner who has an allergy to latex may find the female condom more suitable, as it is made of polyurethane.

12

FEMALE STERILISATION

INTRODUCTION AND HISTORY

Female sterilisation is the only permanent method of female contraception. Today, female sterilisation is performed abdominally by either a mini laparotomy or by laparoscopic sterilisation.

EXPLANATION OF THE METHOD

Female sterilisation involves excising or blocking the fallopian tubes which carry the ovum from the ovary to the uterus. This prevents the ovum from being fertilised by sperm in the fallopian tube.

Efficacy

Female sterilisation is a highly effective form of contraception with a lifetime failure rate of 1 in 200 woman years (FSRH, 2014a). The effectiveness varies depending on which method is used: diathermy and Filshie clips are considered the most effective (FSRH, 2014a).

Disadvantages

- Involves a surgical procedure and anaesthetic
- Not easily reversed

Advantages

- High efficacy
- Permanent
- Effective immediately

Delay the procedure

- Post-partum under six weeks
- Current venous thromboembolism using anti-coagulants

DOI: 10.4324/9781003484424-13

- Major surgery
- Immobility
- Current ischaemic heart disease
- Cervical, ovarian and endometrial cancer
- Current PID or sexually transmitted infection
- Current gallbladder disease

Caution required

- Request for sterilisation at young age, e.g., under 25
- Cerebrovascular accident
- Obesity may be a contraindication for a laparoscopic procedure
- Hypertension
- Epilepsy
- Depressive disorders
- Valvular and congenital heart disease

Range of method

Female sterilisation involves excising or blocking the fallopian tubes as follows:

1 Applying a Hulka-Clemens or Filshie clip – this flattens and occludes the fallopian tube.
2 Drawing up a section of the fallopian tube and applying a Falope ring to the fallopian tube.
3 Excising and ligating the fallopian tube.

Side effects

- If there is a method failure, then there is a higher risk of ectopic pregnancy.
- Feelings of grief and loss.

COUNSELLING A COUPLE FOR FEMALE STERILISATION

Counselling a couple is extremely important for this procedure, as it should be considered a permanent method. Careful counselling will also reduce post-operative regret and grief over the loss of fertility, which some women experience.

During counselling with the couple, you should discuss how they would feel if something happened to their children. How would they feel if something happened to their present partner – would they want children with a new partner? Are they both certain they do not want any more children? There are no set answers to these questions, but they are areas that need to be considered which can be difficult to discuss. It is important to give an unbiased view when discussing sterilisation. You may hold personal views yourself about this method, but these should not influence the couple in their decision. It is useful to meet the couple together, rather than the woman on her own, as the decision affects both parties, and you may get different views and opinions about the decision. However, you may wish to complete the medical history with the woman on her own, as there may be details of her personal medical history that her partner is unaware of, e.g., a previous abortion.

You should complete a full medical history of your client with special attention to gynaecological history. If, for example, she suffers from menorrhagia or dysmenorrhoea, then this will continue following sterilisation. In this situation, it may be more appropriate for her to have the levonorgestrel intrauterine system or have a hysterectomy which would treat these symptoms. In the past, women often complained that a sterilisation caused menorrhagia and dysmenorrhoea; this was more likely due to the fact that once they stopped the combined pill, which had reduced these symptoms, they returned to their true cycle following sterilisation. Research (Rulin et al., 1993) undertaken to investigate the long-term effect of female sterilisation on menses and pelvis pain showed no long-term difference between sterilised and non-sterilised women.

Women should be advised to continue with their present method of contraception until after procedure so that there is no chance of them being pregnant that cycle. If a woman uses an IUD as her method, she should be advised to use condoms for the menstrual cycle prior to the procedure to ensure that no sperm are present in the fallopian tubes, which could fertilise an ovum that is released shortly after surgery, resulting in an ectopic pregnancy.

You should discuss with your clients the efficacy and side effects of sterilisation. Sterilisation is a very effective form of contraception, but if it fails, there is a higher risk of an ectopic pregnancy. You should discuss the difficulties of reversing this procedure so that a couple understands fully the decision they are making. Sterilisation should not be performed at a termination of pregnancy or following childbirth, as the failure rate is higher due to increased vascularity of the tissues involved, and there may also be regret of the decision made at this emotional time.

Procedure

Female sterilisation is usually performed under general or local anaesthetic, and the most common procedure is laparoscopic sterilisation. This is where a small incision is made at the umbilicus, and the abdomen is filled with carbon dioxide gas. The operating table is tilted backwards, which ensures that all the other organs move away from the uterus. Using the laparoscope, the fallopian tubes are located and either ligated or clips applied. This procedure may be performed as a day case and, depending on home circumstances, it may be possible for the woman to go home that day.

If a woman has had previous gynaecological surgery or is obese, it may not be possible to perform a laparoscopic sterilisation. In this situation, a mini laparotomy may be indicated. This procedure involves a larger abdominal incision and usually requires hospitalisation of four to five days. After the sterilisation, most surgeons perform a dilatation and curettage (D&C) to ensure that there is no risk of pregnancy following sexual intercourse prior to the procedure.

Post-female sterilisation

Following the procedure, women may complain of cramp-like period pain for a few days and shoulder pain. This occurs as a result of using carbon dioxide gas and the application of the clips. Women should be advised to continue contraception for seven days post-sterilisation; Cu-IUDs and LNG-IUDs should not be removed until after this time (FSRH, 2014a).

Women should be advised to seek medical attention immediately if they experience any signs of pregnancy or miss a menstrual period. This should be investigated to exclude an intrauterine or extrauterine pregnancy.

Women who experience regret over their decision and signs of grief and loss should be offered post-operative counselling, although counselling prior to the operation should reduce this problem.

Reversal of female sterilisation

Female sterilisation should be considered irreversible. Successful reversal will depend on the type of procedure used when the woman was initially sterilised, her age and the skill of the surgeon performing the reversal. The success in achieving pregnancy following reversal can be between 50% and 90%, depending on the original method used. Following reversal, a woman is at a higher risk of ectopic pregnancy, with 3%–5% of pregnancies being ectopic (Belfield, 1997; FSRH, 2014a).

The methods of sterilisation which are most easily reversed are the use of Hulka or Filshie clips, as these flatten the fallopian tubes, which can be re-inflated. Cautery and diathermy are the hardest to reverse and are used less often these days because of the dangers of damaging other organs. The Falope ring can cause a portion of the fallopian tube to necrose, making reversal more difficult.

SELF-ASSESSMENT QUESTIONS

Answers and discussion at the end of the chapter.

1 Which women do you think are most suitable for female sterilisation?
2 In what way is age relevant to a request for female sterilisation?

SEXUALITY AND ANXIETIES

Women who have a sterilisation often feel liberated – they no longer have the anxiety of pregnancy. Often, a pregnancy scare precipitates a request for sterilisation. This newfound freedom from anxiety enables many women to explore their own sexuality and allow them to enjoy sexual intercourse in a way they have been unable to do before.

ANSWERS TO SELF-ASSESSMENT QUESTIONS

1   Which women do you think are most suitable for a female sterilisation?

Women who are most suitable for sterilisation are those who have completed their families and are in stable relationships. They have considered their future and thought carefully about all the options available to them.

2   In what way is age relevant to a request for female sterilisation?

If a woman is under the age of 30, then a request for sterilisation needs to be treated with caution. There will be concern that a woman may change her mind and want to have more children, especially if something happens to her present relationship.

Women who are older, in their 40s, may have only a few fertile years left. It may be more appropriate for these women to choose a long-acting reversible contraceptive method with a high efficacy like the progestogen implant or injectable, or the LNG-IUD or Cu-IUD. Often, women have not considered these methods.

PREGNANCY: WANTED AND UNWANTED, AND PRECONCEPTUAL CARE

13

INTRODUCTION

Pregnancy is an area of great concern for women who attend for contraception and sexual health advice. Women may consult concerned that they are unable to become pregnant; this may be connected to guilt over previous genitourinary infections or terminations of pregnancy or anxiety over using a method of contraception for a prolonged period like the combined oral contraceptive. Other women may consult unaware that they are at risk of pregnancy, and this topic may need to be approached. Some women may already be aware that they are pregnant and require confirmation; they may have decided about the future of their pregnancy. Other women may need time to consider their decision and discuss this with their partner.

If there is any suspicion that a woman may be pregnant, a pregnancy test should be performed to confirm this. Sometimes a woman can be so adamant that she is not pregnant that when a pregnancy test disproves this, she can find it hard to believe the test results. A pregnancy test should be performed one week after a missed period or three weeks after an episode of unprotected sexual intercourse. It is useful to take a history, which should include menstrual cycle length and episodes of unprotected sexual intercourse and contraception, along with any symptoms of pregnancy. Often, a woman will tell you openly how she feels about a pregnancy, but if she does not discuss her feelings, it is helpful to approach this subject prior to performing the test, as this will help you when you must give her the results.

ACTIVITY

What abortion facilities are available locally to you? Why not see if you can visit so that you can ensure you are giving up-to-date information?

NEGATIVE PREGNANCY TEST

If a pregnancy test is negative, it may be because the test has been performed too early or because the specimen is too dilute or too old, giving a false negative result.

A false negative result can also be due to an ectopic pregnancy or a miscarriage, which will require further investigation if suspected. Details of menstrual cycle, contraception and any episodes of unprotected sexual intercourse should be ascertained. Any complaints of abdominal pain will necessitate further examination through pelvic ultrasound to exclude an ectopic pregnancy or miscarriage.

POSITIVE PREGNANCY TEST

If a pregnancy test is positive and a woman wishes to continue with the pregnancy, she can usually self-refer to her general practitioner for antenatal care to be organised. However sometimes women are unprepared for a positive result and may need time to discuss this with their partner. An appointment should be made at a convenient time, preferably with you, soon. It is useful to work out the gestation of the pregnancy, as this will give you an idea of when to see your client for a follow-up appointment. You should discuss the options available to her so that she can think and discuss this with her partner. Some women already have a suspicion that they are pregnant and have thought about their options already, basing a decision on their feelings.

It is important to allow a woman time to express her feelings. Many women will ask what you would do in this situation. It is important not to influence a client over her decision and to give non-judgemental counselling. A decision over an unwanted pregnancy is probably one of the hardest dilemmas a woman must face, yet it will in the long term be easier if she has been allowed to make this decision herself; an empathetic approach will help her to do this.

SYMPTOMS OF PREGNANCY

Women may complain of the following symptoms of pregnancy:

- Nausea and vomiting
- Increased micturition
- Amenorrhoea
- Breast changes
- Skin changes

SIGNS OF PREGNANCY

Certain signs help to confirm pregnancy.

- Positive pregnancy test
- Enlarged uterus
- Foetal heart sounds can be heard at ten weeks by Sonicaid ultrasonic equipment
- Foetal movements felt
- Foetal parts felt
- Ultrasound can be used to diagnose pregnancy at six weeks
- X-ray can show foetal skeletons at 14–16 weeks but should be avoided, as irradiation can damage the developing foetus

PREGNANCY COUNSELLING

If a woman feels that she does not want to continue with her pregnancy, she has two main options: she can have the baby adopted or have the pregnancy terminated with an abortion. These days, it is rare for women to choose to have their baby adopted, and most women will opt for an abortion. A total of 214,869 abortions were reported in England and Wales in 2021, the highest rate since the Abortion Act was introduced (DHSC, 2023); 87% of women chose a medical abortion over a surgical abortion. Abortion rates are lowest in women under the age of 18 but are highest in women aged 22 and above (DHSC, 2023). Ninety-nine per cent of abortions were funded by the NHS, so providing and encouraging effective contraceptive use can not only prevent a woman going through an emotional procedure but can save the NHS money. The National Institute of Health and Care Excellence (NICE, 2019) has produced clinical guidelines for induced abortion; these recommend ideally that

- all women are offered an assessment appointment within one week of referral, and
- all women undergo an abortion within one week from the assessment.

Women can choose to have an abortion privately or through the NHS. If they wish to have an abortion via the NHS, they may need to attend their local sexual health clinic or GP for a referral to be made locally. If they choose to have a private abortion, it should be a clinic approved by the Department of Health for this procedure.

It is useful to give women a brief outline about the choices of abortion available. It is safer for a woman and less traumatic to have an abortion before 12 weeks. If a woman chooses to have a private abortion, then an early abortion before 12 weeks will cost less and can be performed as a day case. Women often mistakenly believe that they will have the abortion at the initial consultation. They should be warned that this appointment usually involves the completing of a medical history. Usually, a pregnancy test is repeated, and an ultrasound examination will be performed to confirm gestation and exclude ectopic pregnancy. Women will receive pre-abortion counselling at this appointment, and a date for the abortion procedure will be organised. If at any stage a woman wishes to change her mind about her decision, she can at any point. As it is such a difficult decision, sometimes it does happen, and it is important that she is aware that she has this opportunity.

ACTIVITY

Do you know where women can be referred locally for private and NHS abortions? Do you know how much a private abortion would cost in your area?

An abortion can be carried out under the 1967 Abortion Act if two registered medical doctors find that it is necessary on one or more counts prior to 24 weeks' gestation. These are that if the pregnancy were to continue it would involve risk to the life of the woman or would cause injury to her physical or mental health or would cause injury to existing children's physical or mental health. Lastly, there is a substantial risk of the child being born with physical or mental abnormalities. An amendment to this Act in 1991 reduced the upper limit from 28 to 24 weeks' gestation, but in special circumstances, this limit does not apply. These circumstances are when the life of the woman is at risk or there is a possibility of permanent injury, or when there is serious foetal handicap.

You should encourage your client to return following the procedure for a follow-up appointment so that she can discuss how she feels, and any problems can be approached.

It is a good idea to encourage your client to do a sexually transmitted infection screen for chlamydia and gonorrhoea, HIV and syphilis; this should be performed along with the provision of contraception, and this can be done at the initial consultation. Women may not have considered contraception following the procedure, so it is useful to discuss this and, if possible, provide it so that it can be commenced immediately after the abortion; this will help reduce any anxiety afterwards. Women often say, "Never again," so they are only too happy to discuss contraception and may choose a different method as they may have a loss of confidence if they have had a method failure.

INFORMATION THAT SHOULD BE PROVIDED TO WOMEN REQUESTING AN ABORTION

The RCOG recommends that the following information be given to women requesting an abortion. This should be given in an easy-to-understand way with the safety of the methods emphasised (RCOG, 2015).

- The types of abortions available and what these involve
- The side effects, risks and complications associated with each method
- What will happen during and after the abortion
- What they will experience during and following the abortion, e.g., pain, bleeding
- How long the abortion will take
- How pain will be managed
- Follow-up care
- How women may feel emotionally
- Contraceptive advice and STI screening
- Support for women experiencing sexual coercion or domestic violence

CONTRACEPTION FOLLOWING ABORTION

The diaphragm and cervical cap should be refitted following an abortion in case a new size is required, whilst the Cu-IUD and LNG-IUD can be inserted immediately following a first trimester abortion. Following a termination of pregnancy, the progestogen implant may be inserted immediately; if inserted later, then additional contraception will be required for seven days. The progestogen injectable can be given within the first seven days with no extra precautions required, whilst POPs or combined oral contraceptives should be commenced the same day or next day with no additional precautions required following a first trimester abortion.

METHODS OF ABORTION

The main methods of abortion are as follows:

1) Surgical abortion, which can be carried out by
   a) vacuum aspiration,
   b) dilatation and curettage (D&C), or
   c) dilatation and evacuation (D&E).
2) Medical abortion

SURGICAL ABORTION

Vacuum aspiration

This is where the cervix is dilated under general anaesthetic and the contents of the uterus emptied by suction. This is the most widely used method and is carried out before 12 weeks' gestation, usually as a day case.

DILATATION AND CURETTAGE (D&C)

The cervix is dilated, and a curette is introduced into the uterus and the contents removed. This is usually carried out under general anaesthetic.

DILATATION AND EVACUATION (D&E)

Again, this is performed under general anaesthetic. The cervix is dilated, and the contents of the uterus emptied. Vacuum aspiration is performed after this. This method is usually performed in second trimester abortions and can be undertaken up to 20 weeks, although it is preferable to do this before 16 weeks to reduce the risks of a late abortion.

MEDICAL ABORTION

A medical abortion can be carried out at home if a pregnancy is less than or equal to nine weeks and six days' gestation, which is confirmed by ultrasound scan. If the pregnancy is over 10 weeks, then the medical abortion must be carried out in hospital or a designated clinic. It involves, following counselling, the administration of oral mifepristone tablets on day 1 with an observation period of two hours, if a woman is less than ten weeks gestation, this can be taken at home. If the woman vomits within this period, then she will have to be referred for a surgical abortion. Some women experience vaginal bleeding and period-like abdominal cramps. Abdominal pain should not be treated with non-steroidal anti-inflammatory drugs, e.g., aspirin, ibuprofen, mefenamic acid, but other analgesics may be given. Contact telephone numbers are given. If heavy bleeding or severe pain is experienced, then clients may need to be admitted earlier.

This is followed 24–48 hours later, if under 10 weeks gestation at home, with misoprostol given by the vaginal, buccal or sublingual route. If the woman is over ten weeks gestation, this will happen in a designated clinic or hospital. She is observed for six hours in order to observe blood pressure and any problems which may be experienced. Vaginal bleeding usually begins within two hours after administration and may continue for 12 days, gradually lessening. Women will experience abdominal pain, and the abortion should occur within the six-hour period.

A follow-up and ultrasound should be offered if successful abortion has not been confirmed to exclude continuing pregnancy.

CONTRAINDICATIONS

- Suspected ectopic pregnancy
- Allergy to treatment medication
- Chronic adrenal failure
- Long-term corticosteroid therapy
- Haemorrhagic disorders
- Anti-coagulant treatment
- Smokers aged over 35

RELATIVE CONTRAINDICATIONS

- Asthmatics and chronic obstructive airways disease
- Cardiovascular disease
- Renal or hepatic disease
- Women with prosthetic heart valves

SIDE EFFECTS

Drug-related side effects

- Nausea
- Vomiting
- Diarrhoea
- Faintness
- Hot flashes

Side effects related to treatment

- Infection
- Abdominal pain
- Bleeding

COMPLICATIONS OF ABORTION

- Failure to end pregnancy (risk less than 1 in 100)
- Uterine rupture (risk 1 in 1,000)
- Retained products of conception and surgical intervention (risk less than 5%)

There is no increased risk of placenta praevia, infertility or ectopic pregnancy following abortion; however, there is a small increased risk of preterm birth.

SEXUALITY AND ANXIETIES

An unwanted pregnancy brings many anxieties to women. Even if the decision to have an abortion seems to be right for them, there are inevitably regrets. Women may experience the various stages of grief over their decision-denial, anger, depression and acceptance. How they cope with this loss will depend on the counselling and support they receive. Many women subconsciously remember the date of the abortion and the estimated date of delivery. Often, they expect to be chastised for their mistake by professionals, and caution should be taken over women who wish to have a medical abortion or surgical abortion with local anaesthetic and who feel that in some way they should suffer for their present situation.

Women who have recurrent abortions may be desperately trying to seek help. There may be relationship problems and/or feelings of loss of self-worth underlying their cry for attention. Given time and counselling, these feelings may be able to be approached and explored.

Sometimes women use unplanned pregnancy and abortion to test their relationship, which can cause problems within it. However, it can also bring a couple closer together. Women may become pregnant shortly after their abortion and decide this time to continue with the new pregnancy.

Following an abortion, women may choose to change their method of contraception, as they may feel a loss of faith in it. A review (Hudson & Hawkins, 1995) of contraceptive practices before and after an abortion showed that following an abortion, women changed their method to one with a higher efficacy, generally a hormonal method. Following an abortion, many women have a great deal of anxiety over becoming pregnant again and may consult more with pregnancy scares. Often, clients hold misconceptions about abortion; they may believe that their future fertility is affected, and this can cause a great deal of guilt.

PRECONCEPTUAL CARE

Introduction

Planning a pregnancy involves preconceptual counselling – many women do not think about becoming pregnant before it's too late! It is important to discuss this subject with women prior to conceiving to reduce the incidence of problems in pregnancy. Once a woman is pregnant, she should see her GP for a referral for obstetric care.

Preconceptual care for men

Men wishing to conceive should follow certain guidelines:

Alcohol

Alcohol can damage a man's sperm, making it harder to conceive. Men are recommended to keep consumption low during this period.

Drugs

Illegal drugs can cause problems in conceiving. This is a good time to try and stop through counselling and support.

Smoking

Smoking can affect a man's sperm. This is a good time to stop smoking, as there is an increased risk of cot death if a parent smokes.

Sexually transmitted infections

Screening for sexually transmitted infections should be offered; this should include HIV and syphilis serology, chlamydia and gonorrhoea.

Preconceptual care for women

Women planning to become pregnant should be advised to follow certain guidelines.

Diet

Women should be encouraged to eat a healthy diet low in fat and high in fibre. If they are overweight, they should try to reduce their weight well ahead of conceiving, preferably at least three months beforehand, so that they do not have depleted stores of vitamins and minerals. Women who are underweight may have difficulty conceiving; they should be advised to eat three meals a day, with snacks in between.

Certain foods should be avoided in pregnancy. These include liver, because of its high level of vitamin A, and foods made with uncooked eggs like mayonnaise and undercooked meat because of the risk of salmonella. Cheeses made with unpasteurised milk and mould-ripened cheeses should be avoided, e.g., Brie, Camembert, as they may carry the bacteria *Listeria*, which can lead to miscarriage and stillbirth, and serious illness in the unborn baby. Other foods which should be avoided include pâté and cooked chilled chicken, as these also carry the risk of these infections. Undercooked or raw meat should be avoided, as it increases the risk of contracting toxoplasmosis. Toxoplasmosis is an infection caused by a parasite found in raw or uncooked meat, unpasteurised goat's milk, soil, cat faeces and untreated water.

Alcohol

Alcohol should be avoided in pregnancy to reduce the effects of foetal alcohol syndrome, which causes learning and behavioural problems, poor growth and facial malformations.

Supplements

The Department of Health recommends that women take 400 mcg of folic acid prior to conceiving and until they are 12 weeks pregnant to prevent neural tube defects (Department of Health, 1992).

Toxoplasmosis

This is a parasitic infection which can seriously affect the unborn foetus, causing brain damage and blindness. It is a flu-like illness which is contracted through raw meat, cat faeces and sheep and goat milk. Women should be advised to avoid handling cat litter trays, wash their hands when handling animals and wear gloves when gardening.

Smoking

Smoking should be avoided in pregnancy. It is a good idea to try and give it up prior to pregnancy. Women who smoke in pregnancy are more likely to have a low-birth-weight baby, which is associated with increased mortality and morbidity in the perinatal period and later in infancy (House of Commons Health Committee, 1990–1991).

Rubella and measles, mumps and rubella

It is vital that women are routinely screened for rubella immunity prior to conceiving. If women are susceptible to rubella, then they should be vaccinated. The MMR vaccination requires two doses and will protect against measles, mumps and rubella; pregnancy should be excluded prior to vaccination, and women should avoid pregnancy for one month (BNF, 2023).

If a woman is susceptible to rubella and contracts the disease during the first eight to ten weeks of pregnancy, it can result in congenital rubella syndrome, resulting in damage of 90% of infants. Foetal abnormalities include learning disabilities, cataract, deafness, cardiac abnormalities, intrauterine growth retardation and inflammatory lesion of the brain, lung, liver and bone marrow.

Sickle cell disease and thalassaemia

Women and men who are potential carriers of sickle cell disease and thalassaemia should be routinely screened. Those at risk for sickle cell disease are people of African, West Indian and occasionally of Asian origin, whilst those at risk for thalassaemia are of Mediterranean origin, particularly from Greece, Turkey and Cyprus, and people from Pakistan and India. Screening and genetic counselling can reduce the incidence of these diseases.

Sexually transmitted infections and cervical cytology

Women should be encouraged to sort out any health problems they may have before becoming pregnant. Women should make sure that they have had a recent cervical smear and have had regular dental check-ups. If there is any likelihood of a sexually transmitted infection being present, then full screening should be performed and treatment given. For example, bacterial vaginosis, chlamydia, gonorrhoea and trichomoniasis are all associated with premature labour from premature rupture of membranes and, as a result, low birth weight, so screening can reduce problems in pregnancy.

Medical conditions, drugs and medications

If a woman has a long-term condition such as diabetes or epilepsy or has been advised to avoid pregnancy because of a health condition, she should be encouraged to talk to the medical team caring for her, ideally before she gets pregnant.

However, this may not have happened, as the pregnancy may not be planned, and specialist medical teams will need to be involved early to support pregnancy care.

If a woman is taking illegal drugs, then these are harmful to the foetus. Women taking illegal drugs should try to obtain help and counselling prior to conceiving. If the woman is still using illegal drugs, then she will need referral to specialist teams for support.

Women who are taking legally prescribed drugs should be taken with caution, which is why preconceptual care is important. Drugs that cross the placenta causing congenital malformations are called teratogens. The risk of teratogenicity may increase with the number of medications, for example anti-epileptics. Women who are taking teratogens should have a pregnancy prevention plan in place to reduce the risk of conception (FSRH, 2022). The UK Teratology Information Service website has information on medications which are teratogens https://uktis.org.

Research on medications in pregnancy is unethical and therefore our knowledge of the effects can be limited. Healthcare professionals should ensure that they take a full medication and drug history from women who are planning to get pregnant. If medications that can be bought over the counter are taken, women should check with the pharmacist that these are safe to take at this time.

Useful resources

Information on the safety of medications and drugs can be found from the following:

- https://wwwtoxbase.org. Toxbase is the national poisons information service.
- https://www.uktis.org. UK Teratology Information Service is for health professionals requiring information or to report medication exposures in pregnancy.
- https://www.medicinesinpregnancy.org. Bumps is a website for pregnant women run by the UK Teratology Information Service for information and reporting.

Genetic counselling

Genetic counselling is offered to couples with a personal or family history of an inherited medical condition, e.g., cystic fibrosis or Down's syndrome. This gives couples the opportunity to make an informed decision following discussion of the facts of the condition concerned and risks involved. Genetic counselling involves discussion of the genetic abnormality and appropriate screening. A full history of the couple involved is taken and a family tree developed, which will include the medical history of all family members. From this information, the couple will be given an estimation of the risk to future pregnancies of the disorder occurring, and continued counselling and support will be offered so that they are enabled to come to a decision over future pregnancies.

Screening for inherited blood disorders such as sickle cell disease and thalassemia should be considered. These conditions mainly affect people whose ancestors come from Africa, the Caribbean, the Mediterranean, India, Pakistan, south and Southeast Asia and the Middle East.

Socio-economic influences

Many women become pregnant without seeking advice over health beforehand, whilst only a small minority of women actively seek help and advice in planning a pregnancy. As a result, it is necessary for healthcare professionals to approach the subject of pregnancy with women at an appropriate opportunity. This will not only enable women to make adjustments to their diet and have preconceptual screening but will also give them the time to consider the implications of a pregnancy to their lives. This is particularly important for women who are unable to speak English as their first language, as they may have less access to literature in their own language. It is often unknown if a woman is illiterate, which emphasises the need to discuss issues verbally and how unreliable it is to expect men and women to read literature provided in waiting rooms.

Often, the implications of a pregnancy are not considered until it is too late. In today's financial climate, many couples have debts either to credit cards or in the form of negative equity with their mortgage, or perhaps they are unable to sell a property and are living in a property that is now too small for their family. Many men and women no longer feel that their employment is secure; they may not have a permanent contract with their employer or may have a short-term contract, which may cause them anxiety. It may be that by becoming pregnant, money will be severely restricted, or employment will be at risk; not all employers are sympathetic to pregnancy. Although there is never a perfect time to become pregnant, a couple may be able to make some provisions for a pregnancy if they give time to consider the implications it will make to them now, or they may decide to accept financial hardship or other problems after discussion with each other. By discussing these issues beforehand and negotiating their future, a couple is less likely to have problems within their relationship after the baby is born.

A pregnancy can cement a relationship, making it closer and stronger, but it can also be the final straw to an unsatisfactory one. Sometimes women mistakenly believe that a pregnancy will solve present relationship problems; usually, this is the reverse. Occasionally, there are situations when women have been so desperate to have children, because they see their time running out, that they have failed to look at their long-standing relationship with ignored psychosexual problems, which now have to be approached to achieve a pregnancy.

Today, many women are the "breadwinners" in their families, or their salaries are a major part of the family income. This has put restrictions onto the number of children couples choose to have. Women now delay pregnancy till they are older, and their careers are secure, but this causes many dilemmas as to when the best time for a pregnancy will be. There is of course no 'best time' for a pregnancy, and these need to be explored with clients. It may be that the couple have already left it too late and now have infertility problems, which can cause anger and distress within the relationship at the situation.

Women who are already single parents may be in this situation because of a pregnancy at a young age, a broken relationship, or where women have actively chosen to become pregnant as a single parent. Being a single parent is extremely hard not only for the mother but also for the child involved. Today, men and women live further away from their families, so there is no close-knit family network to help with upbringing of the child, so it all falls on one person.

When counselling men and women about preconceptual issues, your personal views and attitudes should be hidden so that a couple is able to come to their own decision. This can be very difficult as couples will often ask whether you have children or what you would do in the given situation. It is important that their decision is their own, as, however hard this may be, they will be able to accept this more easily in the future if it is their own decision.

Sexuality and anxieties

Today many women delay pregnancy until they are in their 30s or 40s and often fail to think about the implications of this decision. Because contraception is so effective, it has helped to delay the decision of pregnancy, creating a dilemma, as women now have to actively stop contraception to become pregnant. Women may find it harder to become pregnant as they become older, and this can increase their feelings of regret and guilt. Sometimes women find that they have left pregnancy too late, and this can cause a great deal of anguish and heartache. With careful counselling, these feelings may be able to be explored.

REFERENCES

Albert, A.E., Warner, D.L., Hatcher, R.A., Trussell, J. & Bennett, C. (1995) Condom use among female commercial sex workers in Nevada's legal brothels. *American Journal of Public Health* 85:1514–1520.

American Health Consultants. (2000) Femcap in Germany, seeking U.S. approval. *Contraceptive Technology Update* 35–36.

Andersson, K., Odlind, V. & Rybo, G. (1994) Levonorgestrel-releasing and copper releasing (Nova T) IUDs during five years of use: a randomised comparative trial. *Contraception* 49:56–72.

Andersson, K., Mattsson, L-M., Rybo, G. & Stadberg, E. (1992) Intrauterine release of levonorgestrel-a new way of adding progestogen in hormone replacement therapy. *Obstetrics and Gynaecology* 79:963–967.

Bagwell, M.A., Coker, A.L., Thompson, S.J., Baker, E.R. & Addy, C.L. (1995) Primary infertility and oral contraceptive steroid use. *Fertility and Sterility* 63:1161–1166.

Bekele, B. & Fantahun, M. (2012) The standard days method: an addition to the arsenal of family planning method choice in Ethiopia. *Journal of Family Planning Reproductive Healthcare* 38:157–166.

Belfield, T. (1997) *FPA Contraceptive Handbook*, 2nd edition. London: Family Planning Association (FPA).

Birth Control Trust. (1994) Briefing: possible association between abortion and breast cancer. *Letter.*

Black, T. (2003) Comparison of Marie Stopes scalpel and electrocautery no-scalpel vasectomy techniques. *The Journal of Family Planning and Reproductive Sexual Health Care* 29(2):32–34.

BMA, GMSC, HEA, Brook Advisory Centres, FPA & RCGP. (1993) *Joint guidance note: Confidentiality and People under 16.* British Medical Association, General Medical Science Committee, Health Education Authority, Brook Advisory Centres, Family Planning Association and Royal College of General Practitioners.

BNF. (2023) *British National Formulary.* London: BMJ Group and Pharmaceutical Press.

BNF. (2024) *British National Formulary.* London: BMJ Group and Pharmaceutical Press. https://bnf.nice.org.uk/medicines-guidance/guidance-on-prescribing/, accessed 18.4.2024.

Bonn, D. (1996) What prospects for hormonal contraceptives for men? *The Lancet* 347:316.

Bounds, W., Guillebaud, J., Dominik, R. & Dalberth, B. (1995) The diaphragm with and without spermicide. A randomised, comparative efficacy trial. *The Journal of Reproductive Medicine* 40:764–774.

Bounds, W. (1994) Contraceptive efficacy of the diaphragm and cervical caps used in conjunction with a spermicide – a fresh look at the evidence. *The British Journal of Family Planning* 20:84–87.

Bounds, W., Robinson, G., Kubba, A. & Guillebaud, J. (1993) Clinical experience with a levonorgestrel-releasing intrauterine contraceptive device (LNG-IUD) as a contraceptive and in the treatment of menorrhagia. *The British Journal of Family Planning* 19:193–194.

Bounds, W., Guillebaud, J. & Newman, G.B. (1992a) Female condom (Femidom). A clinical study of its use-effectiveness and patient acceptability. *The British Journal of Family Planning* 18:36–41.

Bounds, W., Hutt, S., Kubba, A., Cooper, K., Guillebaud, J. & Newman, G.B. (1992b) Randomised comparative study in 217 women of three disposable plastic IUCD thread retrievers. *British Journal of Obstetrics and Gynaecology* 99:915–919.

Brahams, D. (1995) Medicine and the law: warning about natural reversal of vasectomy. *The Lancet* 345:444.

Canter, A.K. & Goldthorpe, S.B. (1995) Vasectomy – patient satisfaction in general practice: a follow up study. *The British Journal of Family Planning* 21:58–60.

Chantler, E. (1992) Vaginal spermicides: some current concerns. *British Journal of Family Planning* 17:118–119.

Collaborative Group on Hormonal Factors in Breast Cancer. (1996a) Breast cancer and hormonal contraceptives: collaborative reanalysis of individual data on 53 297 women with breast cancer and 100 239 woman without breast cancer from 54 epidemiological studies. *The Lancet* 347:1713–1727.

Collaborative Group on Hormonal Factors in Breast Cancer. (1996b) Breast cancer and hormonal contraceptives. *Contraception* 54:3 (supplement).

Collaborative Study Group on the Desogestrel Progestogen Only Pill. (1998) A double blind study comparing the contraceptive efficacy, acceptability and safety of two progestogen only pills containing desogestrel 75 micrograms/day or Levonorgestrel 30 micrograms/day. *The European Journal of Contraception and Reproductive Health Care* 3:169–178.

CSAC. (1993) Retention of IUDs after the menopause. *British Journal of Family Planning* 18:134–135.

Committee of Safety of Medicines (CSM). (2002) Current problems in pharmacovigilance. *Medicines Control Agency* 28.

Cundy, T., Cornish, J., Evans, M.C., Roberts, H. & Reid, I.R. (1994) Recovery of bone density in women who stop using medroxyprogesterone acetate. *British Medical Journal* 308:247–248.

Cundy, T., Evans, M., Roberts, H., Wattie, D., Ames, R. & Reid, I.R. (1991) Bone density in women receiving depot medroxyprogesterone acetate for contraception. *British Medical Journal* 303:13–16.

Department of Health and Social Care. (2023) *Abortion Statistics in England and Wales: 2021*. London: Crown.

Department of Health. (1992) *Folic Acid and Neural Tube Defects: Guidelines on Prevention*. London: Department of Health (Letter).

Edwardes, J.E. & Moore, A. (1999) Implanon. A review of clinical studies. *Family Planning* 24(4):3–16.

Fifer, H., Saunders, J., Soni, S., Sadiq, S.T. & Fitzgerald, M. (2019) British Association for Sexual Health and HIV national guideline for the management of infection with *Neisseria gonorrhoeae*. *BASHH*. www.bashh.org/guidelines

FSRH. (2025). *FSRH Statement: Ulipristal Acetate and Breastfeeding*. FSRH.

FSRH. (2024a) *FSRH CEU Statement: Mirena® 52mg LNG-IUD: Extension of Licence for Contraception to 8 Years*. Clinical effectiveness unit. FSRH.

FSRH. (2024b) *Service Standards for Vasectomy in Sexual and Reproductive Health Services*. Clinical effectiveness unit. FSRH.

FSRH. (2024c) *FSRH CEU Statement: Response to new study by Roland et al (2024)*. Use of progestogens and the risk of intracranial meningioma: national case-control study. FSRH.

FSRH. (2019 Amended October 2023) *Combined Hormonal Contraception*. Clinical effectiveness unit. FSRH.

FSRH. (2023a) *Intrauterine Contraception*. Clinical effectiveness unit. FSRH.

FSRH. (2023b) *Clinical Guidance: Drug Interactions Between HIV Antiretroviral Therapy (ART) and Contraception*. Clinical effectiveness unit. FSRH.

FSRH. (2023c) *Quick Starting Contraception Clinical Effectiveness Unit*. Faculty of Sexual and Reproductive Healthcare.

FSRH. (2023d) *FSRH CEU Statement: Response to new study by Meaidi et al (2023)*. Venous thromboembolism with use of hormonal contraception and non-steroidal anti-inflammatory drugs: nationwide cohort study 07 September 2023. Faculty of Sexual and Reproductive Healthcare.

FSRH. (2023e) *FSRH CEU Statement: New Manufacturer/MHRA Advice Regarding Nomegestrol Acetate – How Does This Affect Prescribing of Zoely®?* Faculty of Sexual and Reproductive Healthcare.

FSRH. (2023f) *FSRH CEU Statement: We Support Reproductive Justices 'Clap Back On The Contraceptive Patch' Campaign*. Faculty of Sexual and Reproductive Healthcare.

FSRH. (August 2022a amended July 2023) *Progestogen Only Pills*. Clinical effectiveness unit. FSRH.

FSRH. (2022b) *Clinical Guidance: Drug Interactions With Hormonal Contraception Clinical Effectiveness Unit*. Faculty of Sexual and Reproductive Healthcare.

FSRH. (December 2014 amended July 2023) *Progestogen-only Injectable Contraception*. Clinical effectiveness unit. FSRH.

FSRH. (February 2021 amended July 2023) *Progestogen Only Implants*. Clinical effective unit. Faculty of Sexual and Reproductive Healthcare.

FSRH. (March 2017 amended July 2023) *Emergency Contraception Clinical Effectiveness Unit*. Faculty of Sexual and Reproductive Healthcare.

FSRH. (2020) *FSRH CEU Statement: New advice from the MHRA regarding cyproterone acetate: how does this affect prescribing of Co-cyprindiol/Dianette® for acne/hirsutism?* FSRH.

FSRH. (2019a) *Contraceptive Choices For Young People*. Clinical effectiveness unit. FSRH.

FSRH. (2019e) *Overweight, Obesity and Contraception*. Clinical effectiveness unit. FSRH.

FSRH. (2017a) *CEU Statement: Contraceptive Choices And Sexual Health For Transgender And Non-Binary People*. FSRH.

FSRH. (2017b) *Quick Starting Contraception Clinical Effectiveness Unit*. Faculty of Sexual and Reproductive Healthcare.

FSRH. (2016 amended 2019) *UK Medical Eligibility Criteria For Contraceptive Use*. Faculty of Sexual and Reproductive Healthcare.

FSRH. (2015a) *Fertility Awareness Methods*. Clinical effectiveness unit. Faculty of Sexual and Reproductive Healthcare.

FSRH. (2015b) *CEU Statement on Self-administration of Sayana Press*. Clinical effectiveness unit. Faculty of Sexual and Reproductive Healthcare.

FSRH. (2015c) *Barrier Methods For Contraception And STI Prevention*. Clinical effectiveness unit. Faculty of Sexual and Reproductive Healthcare.

FSRH. (2015d) *Intrauterine Contraception*. Clinical effectiveness unit. Faculty of Sexual and Reproductive Healthcare.

FSRH. (2015e) *Problematic Bleeding with Hormonal Contraception*. Clinical Effectiveness Unit. Faculty of Sexual and Reproductive Healthcare.

FSRH. (2014a) *Male and Female Sterilisation*. Clinical effectiveness unit. Faculty of Sexual and Reproductive Healthcare.

FSRH. (2010) *Contraception for Women Aged Over 40 Years*. Clinical effectiveness unit. Faculty of Sexual and Reproductive Healthcare.

FSRH. (2009a) *Management of Unscheduled Bleeding in Women Using Hormonal Contraception*. Faculty of Sexual and Reproductive Healthcare.

FSRH. (2009b) *Combined Vaginal Ring. NuvaRing*. Contraception clinical effectiveness unit. Faculty of Sexual and Reproductive Healthcare.

Faculty of Family Planning and Reproductive Health Care and the Royal College of Obstetricians and Gynaecologists (1996) Statement on hormonal contraceptives and breast cancer, Thursday 20 June 1996, *(Letter)*.

Flynn, A. (1996) Natural family planning. *The British Journal of Family Planning* 21:146–148.

Ford, N. & Mathie, E. (1993) The acceptability and experience of the female condom, Femidom among family planning clinic attenders. *The British Journal of Family Planning* 19:187–192.

FPA. (1995) *FPA Fact File 3B: Contraception: Some Factors Affecting Research and Development*. London: Family Planning Association.

Frezieres, R.G., Walsh, T.L., Nelson, A.L., Clark, V.A. & Coulson, A.H. (1999) Evaluation of the efficacy of a polyurethane condom: results from a randomized, controlled clinical trial. *Family Planning Perspectives* 31(2):81–87.

GARDP. (2023) Positive Results Announced in Largest Pivotal Phase 3 Trial of a First-in-Class Oral Antibiotic to Treat Uncomplicated Gonorrhoea. https://gardp.org/wp-content/uploads/2023/11/Zoliflodacin-Phase-3-Results-Announcement-PressRelease-20231101.pdf, accessed 3.5.2024.

Gbolade, B.A. (2002) Depoprovera and bone density. *The Journal of Family Planning and Reproductive Health Care* 28(1):7–11.

Giovannucci, E., Ascherio, A., Rimm, E., Colditz, G.A., Stampfer, M.J. & Wilett, W.C. (1993a) A prospective cohort study of vasectomy and prostate cancer in US men. *Journal of the American Medical Association* 269:873–877.

Giovannucci, E., Tosteson, T.D., Speizer, F.E., Ascherio, A., Vessey, M.P. & Colditz, G.A. (1993b) A retrospective cohort study of vasectomy and prostate cancer in US men. *Journal of the America Medical Association* 269:878–882.

Gov.UK. (2023a). NHS population screening: information for trans and non-binary people. https://www.gov.uk/government/publications/nhs-population-screening-information-for-transgender-people/nhs-population-screening-information-for-trans-people, accessed 25.6.24.

Gov.UK. (2023b) *Conceptions in England and Wales: 2021*. Conceptions in England and Wales – Office for National Statistics, accessed 3.5.2024.

Gov.UK. (2019) New programme to protect children at risk of exploitation. www.gov.uk/government/news/new-programme-to-protect-children-at-risk-of-exploitation, accessed 11.5.2019.

Gov.UK. (2017) Press release. New crackdown on child groomers comes into force. www.gov.uk/government/news/new-crackdown-on-child-groomers-comes-into-force, accessed 11.5.19.

Guillebaud, J. & Bounds, W. (1983) Control of pain associated with intrauterine device insertion using mefenamic acid. *Research and Clinical Forums* 5:69–74.

Gupta, S. (2016) Challenges in transgender healthcare: the pathology perspective. *American Society for Clinical Pathology* 47(3):180–188.

Hinchliff, J., Tetley, J., Lee, D. & Nazroo, J. (2018). Older adults' experiences of sexual difficulties: Qualitative findings from the English Longitudinal Study of Ageing (ELSA). *Journal of Sex Research* 55(2):152–163.

HM Government. (2016) *Multi-agency Statutory Guidance on Female Genital Mutilation.* Crown Publications. Her Majesty Government.

Home office. (2020) FGM: mandatory reporting in healthcare. https://www.gov.uk/government/publications/mandatory-reporting-of-female-genital-mutilation-procedural-information, accessed 1.5.24.

Hollingworth, B. & Guillebaud, J. (1994) The levonorgestrel intrauterine device. *The Diplomate* 1:247–251.

House of Commons Health Committee (1990–1991) *Maternity Services: Preconception.* London: HMSO (Fourth report, Vol. 1).

Howards, S.S. & Peterson, H.B. (1993) Vasectomy and prostate cancer. Chance, bias or a causal relationship. *Journal of the American Medical Association* 269:913–914.

Hubacher, D., Grimes, D.A. & Gemzell-Danielsson, K. (2013) Pitfalls of research linking the intrauterine device to pelvic inflammatory disease. *Obstet Gynecol* 121:1091–1098.

Hudson, G. & Hawkins, R. (1995) Contraception practices of women attending for termination of pregnancy – a study from South Australia. *The British Journal of Family Planning* 21:61–64.

Ikoni, A. (2002) Efficacy of the levonorgestrel intrauterine system in treating menorrhagia: actualities and ambiguities. *The Journal of Family Planning and Reproduction Health Care* 28(2):99–100.

Indian Council of Medical Research Task Force on Natural Family Planning. (1996) Field trial of billings ovulation method of natural family planning. *Contraception* 53:69–74.

International Family Planning Perspectives. (1992) Invasive cervical cancer risk no greater for DMPA users than for nonusers. *International Family Planning Perspectives* 18:156–157.

Jick, H., Jick, S.S., Gurewich, V., Myers, M.W. & Vasilakis, C. (1995) Risk of idiopathic cardiovascular death and nonfatal venous thromboembolism in women using oral contraceptives with differing progestagen components. *The Lancet* 346:1589–1592.

Knight, J. (2017) *The Complete Guide of Fertility Awareness.* London: Routledge.

Lazorwitz, A., Aquilante, C.L., Oreschak, K., Sheeder, J., Guiahi, M. & Teal, S. (2019) Influence of genetic variants on steady state etonogestrel concentrations among contraceptive implant users. *Obstetrics and Gynaecology.* doi: 10.1097/AOG.0000000000003189

Leiras. (1995) *Mirena Levonorgestrel 20 Micrograms/24 Hours. Product Monograph.* Finland: Leiras.

Marchbanks, P.A., McDonald, J.A., Wilson, H.G., Folger, S.G., Mandel, M.G. & Daling, J.R. (2002) Oral contraceptives and the risk of breast cancer. *New England Journal of Medicine* 346:2025–2032.

Martellozzo, E., Monaghan, A., Adler, J.R., Davidson, J., Leyva, R. & Horvath, M.A.H. (2017) *"I Wasn't Sure It Normal To Watch It". A Quantitative And Qualitative Examination Of The Impact Of Online Pornography On The Values, Attitudes, Beliefs And Behaviours Or Children And Young People*. London: Middlesex University. doi: 10.6084/m9.figshare.3382393

Mascarenhas, L., Newton, P. & Newton, J. (1994) First clinical experience with contraceptive implants in the U.K. *British Journal of Family Planning* 20:60 *(Letter)*.

McCann, M.F. & Potter, L.S. (1994) Progestin-only oral contraception: a comprehensive review. *Contraception* 50:S3–S195.

Mohammed, H. (2018) 100 years of STIs in the UK: a review of national surveillance data. *Sex Trans Infect* 0:1–6.

NHS England. (2023) Clinical guide for front line staff to support the management of patients with a learning disability and autistic people – relevant to all clinical specialties (accessed 3.5.2024).

NICE. (2019) *Abortion Care*. National Institute for Health and Care Excellence.

Nursing and Midwifery Council (NMC). (2015 updated 2018) *The Code. Professional Standards of Practice and Behaviour for Nurses, Midwives and Nursing Associates*. London: The Nursing and Midwifery council.

PARTNER Study Group*. (2019) Risk of HIV transmission through condomless sex in serodifferent gay couples with the HIV-positive partner taking suppressive antiretroviral therapy (PARTNER): final results of a multicentre, prospective, observational study. *The Lancet* 393(10189):2428–2438, DOI: https://doi.org/10.1016/S0140-6736(19)30418-0, accessed 28.1.24.

Pearson, V.A.H., Owen, M.R., Phillips, D.R., Pereira Gray, D.J. & Marshall, M.N. (1995) Pregnant teenagers' knowledge and use of emergency contraception. *British Medical Journal* 310:1644.

Pisake, L. (1994) Depot-medroxyprogesterone acetate (DMPA) and cancer of the endometrium and ovary. *Contraception* 49:203–209.

Rice, C.F., Killick, S.R., Dieben, T. & Coelingh Bennink, H. (1999) A comparison of the inhibition of ovulation achieved by desogestrel 75 micrograms and levonorgestrel 30 micrograms. *Human Reproduction* 14(4):982–985.

Robinson, G.E., Bounds, W., Kubba, A., Judith, A. & Guillebaud, J. (1989) Functional ovarian cysts associated with the levonorgestrel releasing device. *British Journal of Family Planning* 14:131–132.

RCN. (2020a) *Domestic Abuse*. London: RCN.

RCN. (2023) *Domestic Abuse*. London: RCN.

RCN. (2016 updated 2023) *Female Genital Mutilation: An RCN Resource for Nurses and Midwifery Practice*, 3rd edition. London: RCN.

RCN. (2020b) *Fair Care for Trans Patients*, 2ndedition. RCN.

Royal College of Obstetricians and Gynaecologists. (2015) *Best Practice in comprehensive abortion care*. London: RCOG Press. Best practice paper No. 2.

Royal College of Obstetricians and Gynaecologists. (2004) *Male and Female Sterilisation*. London: RCOG Press. Evidence-based Clinical Guideline No 4.

Rulin, M.C., Davidson, A.R., Philliber, S.G., Graves, W.L. & Cushman, L.F. (1993) Long-term effect of tubal sterilization on menstrual indices and pelvic pain. *Obstetrics and Gynaecology* 82:118–121.

Ryder, B. & Campbell, H. (1995) Natural family planning in the 1990s. *The Lancet* 346:233–234.

Simms, M. (1993) Teenage pregnancy – give girls a motive for avoiding it. *British Medical Journal* 306:1749–1750 (*letter*).

Sinai, I., Lundgren, R.I. & Gribble, J.N. (2012) Continued use of the standard days method. *Journal of Family Planning Reproductive Healthcare* 38:150–156.

Sivin, I. & Stern, J. (1994) Health during use of levonorgestrel 20 g/d and the copper TCU 380Ag intrauterine contraceptive devices: a multicenter study. *Fertility and Sterility* 61:70–77.

Smith, T. (1993) Influence of socio economic factors on attaining targets for reducing teenage pregnancies. *British Medical Journal* 306:1232–1235.

Sparrow, M.J. & Lavill, K. (1994) Breakage and slippage of condoms in family planning clients. *Contraception* 50:117–129.

Spitzer, W.O., Lewis, M.A., Heinemann, L.A.J., Thorogood, M. & Macrae, K.D. (1996) Third generation oral contraceptives and risk of venous thrombo-embolic disorders: an international case-control study. *British Medical Journal* 312:83–88.

UK Family Planning Research Network. (1993) Mishaps occurring during condom use, and the subsequent use of post-coital contraception. *British Journal of Family Planning* 19:218–220.

UK Health Security Agency (UKHSA). (2023) Decline in HIV transmission but progress slow in women. https://www.gov.uk/government/news/decline-in-hiv-transmission-but-progress-slow-in-women?mc_cid=d1494aa498&mc_eid=fa47b6d9c9, accessed 3.5.2024.

Vessey, M.P., Yeates, D. & Flynn, S. (2010) Factors affecting mortality in a large cohort study with special reference to oral contraceptive use. *Contraception* 82:221–229.

Vessey, M.P. (1988) Urinary tract infection and the diaphragm. *British Journal of Family Planning* 13:41–43.

West, R.R. (1992) Vasectomy and testicular cancer – no association on current evidence. *British Medical Journal* 304:729–730.

WHO. (1995) World Health Organization collaborative study of cardiovascular disease and steroid hormone contraception. Venous thromboembolic disease and combined oral contraceptives: results of international multicentre case control study. *The Lancet* 346:1575–1581.

WHO. (1992) World health organization collaborative study of neoplasia and steroid contraceptives. Depot medroxyprogesterone acetate (DMPA) and risk of invasive squamous cell cervical cancer. *Contraception* 45:299–312.

WHO. (1991) World health organization collaborative study of neoplasia and steroid contraceptives. Breast cancer and depot-medroxyprogesterone acetate: a multinational study. *The Lancet* 338:833–838.

Wilson, E. (1993) Depoprovera: underused and undervalued. *British Medical Journal* 18:101.

World Health Organisation (WHO). (2024) Classification of female genital mutilation. https://www.who.int/news-room/fact-sheets/detail/female-genital-mutilation, accessed 1.5.2024.

Ziebland, S., Maxwell, K. & Greenhall, E. (1996) 'It's a mega dose of hormones, isn't it?' Why women may be reluctant to use emergency contraception. *British Journal of Family Planning* 22:84–86.

INDEX

Pages in *italics* refer to figures and pages in **bold** refer to tables.

Printed in the United States
by Baker & Taylor Publisher Services